The Intermediate Sex

by

Edward Carpenter (1844-1929)

The Echo Library 2007

Published by

The Echo Library

Echo Library
131 High St.
Teddington
Middlesex TW11 8HH

www.echo-library.com

Please report serious faults in the text to complaints@echo-library.com

ISBN 978-1-40682-381 3

A Study of Some Transitional Types of Men and Women (1908)

"There are transitional forms between the metals and non-metals; between chemical combinations and simple mixtures, between animals and plants, between phanerogams and cryptogams, and between mammals and birds. . . . The improbability may henceforth be taken for granted of finding in Nature a sharp cleavage between all that is masculine on the one side and all that is feminine on the other; or that any living being is so simple in this respect that it can be put wholly on one side, or wholly on the other, of the line."

O. WEININGER.

PREFATORY NOTE

The following papers, now collected in book-form, have been written— and some of them published—on various occasions during the last twelve or fourteen years, and in the intervals of other work; and this must be my excuse for occasional repetitions or overlapping of matter, which may be observable among them. I have thought it best, however, to leave them as they stand, as in this way each is more complete in itself. The second essay, which gives its title to the book, has already appeared in my "Love's Coming-of-Age" (edition 1906), but is reprinted here as belonging more properly to this volume. A collection of quotations from responsible writers, who touch on various sides of the subject, is added at the end, to form an Appendix—which the author thinks will prove helpful, though he does not necessarily endorse all the opinions presented.

E. C.

I

INTRODUCTORY

The subject dealt with in this book is one of great, and one may say growing, importance. Whether it is that the present period is one of large increase in the numbers of men and women of an intermediate or mixed temperament, or whether it merely is that it is a period in which more than usual attention happens to be accorded to them, the fact certainly remains that the subject has great actuality and is pressing upon us from all sides. It is recognised that anyhow the number of persons occupying an intermediate position between the two sexes is very great, that they play a considerable part in general society, and that they necessarily present and embody many problems which, both for their own sakes and that of society, demand solution. The literature of the question has in consequence already grown to be very extensive, especially on the Continent, and includes a great quantity of scientific works, medical treatises, literary essays, romances, historical novels, poetry, etc. And it is now generally admitted that some knowledge and enlightened understanding of the subject is greatly needed for the use of certain classes—as, for instance, medical men, teachers, parents, magistrates, judges, and the like.

That there are distinctions and gradations of Soul-material in relation to Sex—that the inner psychical affections and affinities shade off and graduate, in a vast number of instances, most subtly from male to female, and not always in obvious correspondence with the outer bodily sex—is a thing evident enough to anyone who considers the subject; nor could any good purpose well be served by ignoring this fact—even if it were possible to do so. It is easy of course (as some do) to classify all these mixed or intermediate types as BAD. It is also easy (as some do) to argue that just because they combine opposite qualities they are likely to be GOOD and valuable. But the subtleties and complexities of Nature cannot be despatched in this off-hand manner. The great probability is that, as in any other class of human beings, there will be among these too, good and bad, high and low, worthy and unworthy— some perhaps exhibiting through their double temperament a rare and beautiful flower of humanity, others a perverse and tangled ruin.

Before the facts of Nature we have to preserve a certain humility and reverence; nor rush in with our preconceived and obstinate assumptions. Though these gradations of human type have always, and among all peoples, been more or less known and recognised, yet their frequency to-day, or even the concentration of attention on them, may be the indication of some important change actually in progress. We do NOT know, in fact, what possible evolutions are to come, or what new forms, of permanent place and value, are being already slowly differentiated from the surrounding mass of humanity. It may be that, as at some past period of evolution the worker-bee was without doubt differentiated from the two ordinary bee-sexes, so at the present time certain new types of human kind may be emerging, which will have an important part to play in the societies of the future—even though for the moment their appearance is attended by a good deal of confusion and misapprehension. It may be so; or it may not. We do not know; and the best attitude we can adopt is one of sincere and dispassionate observation of facts.

Of course wherever this subject touches on the domain of love we may expect difficult queries to arise. Yet it is here probably that the noblest work of the intermediate sex or sexes will be accomplished, as well as the greatest errors committed. It seems almost a law of Nature that new and important movements should be misunderstood and vilified—even though afterwards they may be widely approved or admitted to honour. Such movements are always envisaged first from whatever aspect they may possibly present, of ludicrous or contemptible. The early Christians, in the eyes of Romans, were chiefly known as the perpetrators of obscure rites and crimes in the darkness of the catacombs. Modern Socialism was for a long time supposed to be an affair of daggers and dynamite; and even now there are thousands of good people ignorant enough to believe that it simply means "divide up all round, and each take his threepenny bit." Vegetarians were supposed to be a feeble and brainless set of cabbage-eaters. The Women's movement, so vast in its scope and importance, was nothing but an absurd attempt to make women "the apes of men." And so on without end; the accusation in each case being some tag or last fag-end of fact, caught up by ignorance, and coloured by prejudice. So commonplace is it to misunderstand, so easy to misrepresent.

That the Uranian temperament, especially in regard to its affectional side, is not without faults must naturally be allowed; but that it has been grossly and absurdly misunderstood is certain. With a good deal of experience in the matter, I think one may safely say that the defect of the male Uranian, or Urning,[1] is NOT sensuality—but rather SENTIMENTALITY. The lower, more ordinary types of Urning are often terribly sentimental; the superior types strangely, almost incredibly emotional; but neither AS A RULE (though of course there must be exceptions) are so sensual as the average normal man.

This immense capacity of emotional love represents of course a great driving force. Whether in the individual or in society, love is eminently creative. It is their great genius for attachment which gives to the best Uranian types their penetrating influence and activity, and which often makes them beloved and accepted far and wide even by those who know nothing of their inner mind. How many so-called philanthropists of the best kind (we need not mention names) have been inspired by the Uranian temperament, the world will probably never know. And in all walks of life the great number and influence of folk of this disposition, and the distinguished place they already occupy, is only realised by those who are more or less behind the scenes. It is probable also that it is this genius for emotional love which gives to the Uranians their remarkable YOUTHFULNESS.

Anyhow, with their extraordinary gift for, and experience in, affairs of the heart—from the double point of view, both of the man and of the woman—it is not difficult to see that these people have a special work to do as reconcilers and interpreters

---

[1] [Note: For the derivation of these terms see ch. ii., p. 20, intra.]

of the two sexes to each other. Of this I have spoken at more length below (chaps. ii. and v.). It is probable that the superior Urnings will become, in affairs of the heart, to a large extent the teachers of future society; and if so, that their influence will tend to the realisation and expression of an attachment less exclusively sensual than the average of to-day, and to the diffusion of this in all directions.

While at any rate not presuming to speak with authority on so difficult a subject, I plead for the necessity of a patient consideration of it, for the due recognition of the types of character concerned, and for some endeavour to give them their fitting place and sphere of usefulness in the general scheme of society.

One thing more by way of introductory explanation. The word Love is commonly used in so general and almost indiscriminate a fashion as to denote sometimes physical instincts and acts, and sometimes the most intimate and profound feelings; and in this way a good deal of misunderstanding is caused. In this book (unless there be exceptions in the Appendix) the word is used to denote the inner devotion of one person to another; and when anything else is meant— as, for instance, sexual relations and actions— this is clearly stated and expressed.

II

THE INTERMEDIATE SEX

"Urning men and women, on whose book of life Nature has written her new word which sounds so strange to us, bear such storm and stress within them, such ferment and fluctuation, so much complex material having its outlet only towards the future; their individualities are so rich and many-sided, and withal so little understood, that it is impossible to characterise them adequately in a few sentences."—Otto de Joux.

In late years (and since the arrival of the New Woman amongst us) many things in the relation of men and women to each other have altered, or at any rate become clearer. The growing sense of equality in habits and customs—university studies, art, music, politics, the bicycle, etc.—all these things have brought about a rapprochement between the sexes. If the modern woman is a little more masculine in some ways than her predecessor, the modern man (it is to be hoped), while by no means effeminate, is a little more sensitive in temperament and artistic in feeling than the original John Bull. It is beginning to be recognised that the sexes do not or should not normally form two groups hopelessly isolated in habit and feeling from each other, but that they rather represent the two poles of ONE group—which is the human race; so that while certainly the extreme specimens at either pole are vastly divergent, there are great numbers in the middle region who (though differing corporeally as men and women) are by emotion and temperament very near to each other.[2] We all know women with a strong dash of the masculine temperament, and we all know men whose almost feminine sensibility and intuition seem to belie their bodily form. Nature, it might appear, in mixing the elements which go to compose each individual, does not always keep her two groups of

---

[2] [Note: See Appendix.]

ingredients—which represent the two sexes—properly apart, but often throws them crosswise in a somewhat baffling manner, now this way and now that; yet wisely, we must think—for if a severe distinction of elements were always maintained the two sexes would soon drift into far latitudes and absolutely cease to understand each other. As it is, there are some remarkable and (we think) indispensable types of character in whom there is such a union or balance of the feminine and masculine qualities that these people become to a great extent the interpreters of men and women to each other.

There is another point which has become clearer of late. For as people are beginning to see that the sexes form in a certain sense a continuous group, so they are beginning to see that Love and Friendship—which have been so often set apart from each other as things distinct—are in reality closely related and shade imperceptibly into each other. Women are beginning to demand that Marriage shall mean Friendship as well as Passion; that a comrade- like Equality shall be included in the word Love; and it is recognised that from the one extreme of a "Platonic" friendship (generally between persons of the same sex) up to the other extreme of passionate love (generally between persons of opposite sex) no hard and fast line can at any point be drawn effectively separating the different kinds of attachment. We know, in fact, of Friendships so romantic in sentiment that they verge into love; we know of Loves so intellectual and spiritual that they hardly dwell in the sphere of Passion.

A moment's thought will show that the general conceptions indicated above—if anywhere near the truth—point to an immense diversity of human temperament and character in matters relating to sex and love; but though such diversity has probably always existed, it has only in comparatively recent times become a subject of study. More than thirty years ago, however, an Austrian writer, K. H. Ulrichs, drew attention in a series of pamphlets (Memnon, Ara Spei, Inclusa, etc.) to the existence of a class of people who strongly illustrate the above remarks, and with whom specially this paper is concerned. He pointed out that there were people born in such a position—as it were on the dividing line between the sexes— that while belonging distinctly to one sex as far as their bodies are concerned they may be said to belong MENTALLY and EMOTIONALLY to the other; that there were men, for instance, who might be described as of feminine soul enclosed in a male body (anima muliebris in corpore virili inclusa), or in other cases, women whose definition would be just the reverse. And he maintained that this doubleness of nature was to a great extent proved by the special direction of their love-sentiment. For in such cases, as indeed might be expected, the (apparently) masculine person instead of forming a love-union with a female tended to contract romantic friendships with one of his own sex; while the apparently feminine would, instead of marrying in the usual way, devote herself to the love of another feminine.

People of this kind (i.e., having this special variation of the love-sentiment) he called Urnings;[3] and though we are not obliged to accept his theory about the crosswise connexion between "soul" and "body," since at best these words are somewhat vague and indefinite; yet his work was important because it was one of the first attempts, in modern times, to recognise the existence of what might be called an Intermediate sex, and to give at any rate SOME explanation of it. [4]Since that

---

[3] [Note: Charles G. Leland ("Hans Breitmann") in his book "The Alternate Sex" (Wellby, 1904), insists much on the frequent combination of the characteristics of both sexes in remarkable men and women, and has a chapter on "The Female Mind in Man," and another on "The Male Intellect in Woman."]

[4] [Note: Charles G. Leland ("Hans Breitmann") in his book "The Alternate Sex" (Wellby, 1904), insists much on the frequent combination of the characteristics of both sexes in remarkable men and women, and has a chapter on "The Female Mind in Man," and another on "The Male Intellect in Woman."]

time the subject has been widely studied and written about by scientific men and others, especially on the Continent (though in England it is still comparatively unknown), and by means of an extended observation of present-day cases, as well as the indirect testimony of the history and literature of past times, quite a body of general conclusions has been arrived at—of which I propose in the following pages to give some slight account.

Contrary to the general impression, one of the first points that emerges from this study is that "Urnings," or Uranians, are by no means so very rare; but that they form, beneath the surface of society, a large class. It remains difficult, however, to get an exact statement of their numbers; and this for more than one reason: partly because, owing to the want of any general understanding of their case, these folk tend to conceal their true feelings from all but their own kind, and indeed often deliberately act in such a manner as to lead the world astray— (whence it arises that a normal man living in a certain society will often refuse to believe that there is a single Urning in the circle of his acquaintance, while one of the latter, or one that understands the nature, living in the same society, can count perhaps a score or more)—and partly because it is indubitable that the numbers do vary very greatly, not only in different countries but even in different classes in the same country. The consequence of all this being that we have estimates differing very widely from each other. Dr. Grabowsky, a well-known writer in Germany, quotes figures (which we think must be exaggerated) as high as one man in every 22, while Dr. Albert Moll (Die Conträre Sexualempfindung, chap. 3) gives estimates varying from 1 in every 50 to as low as 1 in every 500. [5]These figures apply to such as are exclusively of the said nature, i.e., to those whose deepest feelings of love and friendship go out only to persons of their own sex. Of course, if in addition are included those double-natured people (of whom there is a great number) who experience the normal attachment, with the

---

[5] [Note: Some late statistical inquiries (see Statistische Untersuchungen, by Dr. M. Hirschfeld, Leipzig, 1904) yield 1.5 to 2.0 per cent. as a probable ratio. See also Appendix,]

homogenic tendency in less or greater degree superadded, the estimates must be greatly higher.

In the second place it emerges (also contrary to the general impression) that men and women of the exclusively Uranian type are by no means necessarily morbid in any way—unless, indeed, their peculiar temperament be pronounced in itself morbid. Formerly it was assumed, as a matter of course, that the type was merely a result of disease and degeneration; but now with the examination of the actual facts it appears that, on the contrary, many are fine, healthy specimens of their sex, muscular and well- developed in body, of powerful brain, high standard of conduct, and with nothing abnormal or morbid of any kind observable in their physical structure or constitution. This is of course not true of all, and there still remain a certain number of cases of weakly type to support the neuropathic view. Yet it is very noticeable that this view is much less insisted on by the later writers than by the earlier. It is also worth noticing that it is now acknowledged that even in the most healthy cases the special affectional temperament of the "Intermediate" is, as a rule, ineradicable; so much so that when (as in not a few instances) such men and women, from social or other considerations, have forced themselves to marry and even have children, they have still not been able to overcome their own bias, or the leaning after all of their life-attachment to some friend of their own sex.

This subject, though obviously one of considerable interest and importance, has been hitherto, as I have pointed out, but little discussed in this country, partly owing to a certain amount of doubt and distrust which has, not unnaturally perhaps, surrounded it. And certainly if the men and women born with the tendency in question were only exceedingly rare, though it would not be fair on that account to ignore them, yet it would hardly be necessary to dwell at great length on their case. But as the class is really, on any computation, numerous, it becomes a duty for society not only to understand them but to help them to understand themselves.

For there is no doubt that in many cases people of this kind suffer a great deal from their own temperament—and yet, after all, it is possible that they may have an important part to play in

14

the evolution of the race. Anyone who realises what Love is, the dedication of the heart, so profound, so absorbing, so mysterious, so imperative, and always just in the noblest natures so strong, cannot fail to see how difficult, how tragic even, must often be the fate of those whose deepest feelings are destined from the earliest days to be a riddle and a stumbling-block, unexplained to themselves, passed over in silence by others. [6]To call people of such temperament "morbid," and so forth, is of no use. Such a term is, in fact, absurdly inapplicable to many, who are among the most active, the most amiable and accepted members of society; besides, it forms no solution of the problem in question, and only amounts to marking down for disparagement a fellow-creature who has already considerable difficulties to contend with. Says Dr. Moll, "Anyone who has seen many Urnings will probably admit that they form a by no means enervated human group; on the contrary, one finds powerful, healthy-looking folk among them;" but in the very next sentence he says that they "suffer severely" from the way they are regarded; and in the manifesto of a considerable community of such people in Germany occur these words, "The rays of sunshine in the night of our existence are so rare, that we are responsive and deeply grateful for the least movement, for every single voice that speaks in our favour in the forum of mankind." [7]In dealing with this class of folk, then, while I do not deny that they present a difficult problem, I think that just for that very reason their case needs discussion. It would be a great mistake to suppose that their attachments are necessarily sexual, or connected with sexual acts. On the contrary (as abundant evidence shows), they are often purely emotional in their character; and to confuse Uranians (as is so often done) with libertines having no law but curiosity in self-indulgence is to do them a great wrong. At the same time, it is evident that their special temperament may sometimes cause them difficulty in regard to their sexual

---

[6] [Note: For instances, see Appendix]

[7] [Note: See De Joux, Die Enterbten des Liebesglückes (Leipzig, 1893), p. 21.]

relations. Into this subject we need not just now enter. But we may point out how hard it is, especially for the young among them, that a veil of complete silence should be drawn over the subject, leading to the most painful misunderstandings, and perversions and confusions of mind; and that there should be no hint of guidance; nor any recognition of the solitary and really serious inner struggles they may have to face! If the problem is a difficult one—as it undoubtedly is—the fate of those people is already hard who have to meet it in their own persons, without their suffering in addition from the refusal of society to give them any help. It is partly for these reasons, and to throw a little light where it may be needed, that I have thought it might be advisable in this paper simply to give a few general characteristics of the Intermediate types.

As indicated then already, in bodily structure there is, as a rule, nothing to distinguish the subjects of our discussion from ordinary men and women; but if we take the general mental characteristics it appears from almost universal testimony that the male tends to be of a rather gentle, emotional disposition— with defects, if such exist, in the direction of subtlety, evasiveness, timidity, vanity, etc.; while the female is just the opposite, fiery, active, bold and truthful, with defects running to brusqueness and coarseness. Moreover, the mind of the former is generally intuitive and instinctive in its perceptions, with more or less of artistic feeling; while the mind of the latter is more logical, scientific, and precise than usual with the normal woman. So marked indeed are these general characteristics that sometimes by means of them (though not an infallible guide) the nature of the boy or girl can be detected in childhood, before full development has taken place; and needless to say it may often be very important to be able to do this.

It was no doubt in consequence of the observation of these signs that K. H. Ulrichs proposed his theory; and though the theory, as we have said, does not by any means meet ALL the facts, still it is perhaps not without merit, and may be worth bearing in mind.

In the case, for instance, of a woman of this temperament (defined we suppose as "a male soul in a female body") the theory helps us to understand how it might be possible for her to fall bonâ fide in love with another woman. Krafft-Ebing gives [8]the case of a lady (A.), 28 years of age, who fell deeply in love with a younger one (B.). "I loved her divinely," she said. They lived together, and the union lasted four years, but was then broken by the marriage of B. A. suffered in consequence from frightful depression; but in the end—though without real love—got married herself. Her depression however only increased and deepened into illness. The doctors, when consulted, said that all would be well if she could only have a child. The husband, who loved his wife sincerely, could not understand her enigmatic behaviour. She was friendly to him, suffered his caresses, but for days afterwards remained "dull, exhausted, plagued with irritation of the spine, and nervous." Presently a journey of the married pair led to another meeting with the female friend—who had now been wedded (but also unhappily) for three years. "Both ladies trembled with joy and excitement as they fell into each other's arms, and were thenceforth inseparable. The man found that this friendship relation was a singular one, and hastened the departure. When the opportunity occurred, he convinced himself from the correspondence between his wife and her 'friend' that their letters were exactly like those of two lovers."

It appears that the loves of such women are often very intense, and (as also in the case of male Urnings) life-long. [9]Both classes feel themselves blessed when they love happily. Nevertheless, to many of them it is a painful fact that—in consequence of their peculiar temperament—they are, though fond of children, not in the position to found a family.

We have so far limited ourselves to some very general characteristics of the Intermediate race. It may help to clear and fix our ideas if we now describe in more detail, first, what may be called the extreme and exaggerated types of the race, and then the more normal and perfect types. By doing so we shall get a more definite and concrete view of our subject.

---

[8] [Note: "Psychopathia Sexualis," 7th ed., p. 276.]
[9] [Note: See Appendix.]

In the first place, then, the extreme specimens—as in most cases of extremes—are not particularly attractive, sometimes quite the reverse. In the male of this kind we have a distinctly effeminate type, sentimental, lackadaisical, mincing in gait and manners, something of a chatterbox, skilful at the needle and in woman's work, sometimes taking pleasure in dressing in woman's clothes; his figure not unfrequently betraying a tendency towards the feminine, large at the hips, supple, not muscular, the face wanting in hair, the voice inclining to be high-pitched, etc.; while his dwelling- room is orderly in the extreme, even natty, and choice of decoration and perfume. His affection, too, is often feminine in character, clinging, dependent and jealous, as of one desiring to be loved almost more than to love. [10]

On the other hand, as the extreme type of the homogenic female, we have a rather markedly aggressive person, of strong passions, masculine manners and movements, practical in the conduct of life, sensuous rather than sentimental in love, often untidy, and outré in attire;[11] her figure muscular, her voice rather low in pitch; her dwelling-room decorated with sporting-scenes, pistols, etc., and not without a suspicion of the fragrant weed in the atmosphere; while her love (generally to rather soft and feminine specimens of her own sex) is often a sort of furor, similar to the ordinary masculine love, and at times almost uncontrollable.

These are types which, on account of their salience, everyone will recognise more or less. Naturally, when they occur they excite a good deal of attention, and it is not an uncommon impression that most persons of the homogenic nature belong to either one or other of these classes. But in

---

[10] [Note: A good deal in this description may remind readers of history of the habits and character of Henry III. of France.]

[11] [Note: Perhaps, like Queen Christine of Sweden, who rode across Europe, on her visit to Italy, in jack- boots and sitting astride of her horse. It is said that she shook the Pope's hand, on seeing him, so heartily that the doctor had to attend to it afterwards!]

reality, of course, these extreme developments are rare, and for the most part the temperament in question is embodied in men and women of quite normal and unsensational exterior. Speaking of this subject and the connection between effeminateness and the homogenic nature in men, Dr. Moll says: "It is, however, as well to point out at the outset that effeminacy does not by any means show itself in all Urnings. Though one may find this or that indication in a great number of cases, yet it cannot be denied that a very large percentage, perhaps by far the majority of them, do NOT exhibit pronounced Effeminacy." And it may be supposed that we may draw the same conclusion with regard to women of this class—namely, that the majority of them do not exhibit pronounced masculine habits. In fact, while these extreme cases are of the greatest value from a scientific point of view as marking tendencies and limits of development in certain directions, it would be a serious mistake to look upon them as representative cases of the whole phases of human evolution concerned.

If now we come to what may be called the more normal type of the Uranian man, we find a man who, while possessing thoroughly masculine powers of mind and body, combines with them the tenderer and more emotional soul-nature of the woman—and sometimes to a remarkable degree. Such men, as said, are often muscular and well- built, and not distinguishable in exterior structure and the carriage of body from others of their own sex; but emotionally they are extremely complex, tender, sensitive, pitiful and loving, "full of storm and stress, of ferment and fluctuation" of the heart; the logical faculty may or may not, in their case, be well-developed, but intuition is always strong; like women they read characters at a glance, and know, without knowing how, what is passing in the minds of others; for nursing and waiting on the needs of others they have often a peculiar gift; at the bottom lies the artist-nature, with the artist's sensibility and perception. Such an one is often a dreamer, of brooding, reserved habits, often a musician, or a man of culture, courted in society, which nevertheless does not understand him—though sometimes a child of the people, without any culture, but almost always with a peculiar inborn refinement. De Joux, who speaks on the whole favourably of

Uranian men and women, says of the former: "They are enthusiastic for poetry and music, are often eminently skilful in the fine arts, and are overcome with emotion and sympathy at the least sad occurrence. Their sensitiveness, their endless tenderness for children, their love of flowers, their great pity for beggars and crippled folk are truly womanly." And in another passage he indicates the artist-nature, when he says: "The nerve- system of many an Urning is the finest and the most complicated musical instrument in the service of the interior personality that can be imagined."

It would seem probable that the attachment of such an one is of a tender and profound character; indeed, it is possible that in this class of men we have the love sentiment in one of its most perfect forms—a form in which from the necessities of the situation the sensuous element, though present, is exquisitely subordinated to the spiritual. Says one writer on this subject, a Swiss, "Happy indeed is that man who has won a real Urning for his friend—he walks on roses, without ever having to fear the thorns"; and he adds, "Can there ever be a more perfect sick-nurse than an Urning?" And though these are ex parte utterances, we may believe that there is an appreciable grain of truth in them. Another writer, quoted by De Joux, speaks to somewhat the same effect, and may perhaps be received in a similar spirit. "We form," he says, "a peculiar aristocracy of modest spirits, of good and refined habit, and in many masculine circles are the representatives of the higher mental and artistic element. In us dreamers and enthusiasts lies the continual counterpoise to the sheer masculine portion of society—inclining, as it always does, to mere restless greed of gain and material sensual pleasures."

That men of this kind despise women, though a not uncommon belief, is one which hardly appears to be justified. Indeed, though naturally not inclined to "fall in love" in this direction, such men are by their nature drawn rather near to women, and it would seem that they often feel a singular appreciation and understanding of the emotional needs and destinies of the other sex, leading in many cases to a genuine though what is called "Platonic" friendship. There is little doubt that they are often instinctively sought after by women, who, without suspecting the real cause, are conscious of a sympathetic chord in the homogenic which they miss in the normal man. To quote De Joux once more: "It would be a mistake to suppose that all Urnings must be woman-haters. Quite the contrary. They are not seldom the faithfulest friends, the truest allies, and most convinced defenders of women."

To come now to the more normal and perfect specimens of the homogenic WOMAN, we find a type in which the body is thoroughly feminine and gracious, with the rondure and fulness of the female form, and the continence and aptness of its movements, but in which the inner nature is to a great extent masculine; a temperament active, brave, originative, somewhat decisive, not too emotional; fond of out-door life, of games and sports, of science, politics, or even business; good at organisation, and well-pleased with positions of responsibility, sometimes indeed making an excellent and generous leader. Such a woman, it is easily seen, from her special combination of qualities, is often fitted for remarkable work, in professional life, or as manageress of institutions, or even as ruler of a country. Her love goes out to younger and more feminine natures than her own; it is a powerful passion, almost of heroic type, and capable of inspiring to great deeds; and when held duly in leash may sometimes become an invaluable force in the teaching and training of girl-hood, or in the creation of a school of thought or action among women. Many a Santa Clara, or abbess-founder of religious houses, has probably been a woman of this type; and in all times such women—not being bound to men by the ordinary ties—have been able to work the more freely for the interests of their sex, a cause to which their own temperament impels them to devote themselves con amore.

I have now sketched—very briefly and inadequately it is true—both the extreme types and the more healthy types of the "Intermediate" man and woman: types which can be verified from history and literature, though more certainly and satisfactorily perhaps from actual life around us. And unfamiliar though the subject is, it begins to appear that it is one which modern thought and science will have to face. Of the latter and more normal types it may be said that they exist, and have always existed, in considerable abundance, and from that circumstance alone there is a strong probability that they have their place and purpose. As pointed out there is no particular indication of morbidity about them, unless the special nature of their love-sentiment be itself accounted morbid; and in the alienation of the sexes from each other, of which complaint is so often made to-day, it must be admitted that they do much to fill the gap.

The instinctive artistic nature of the male of this class, his sensitive spirit, his wavelike emotional temperament, combined with hardihood of intellect and body; and the frank, free nature of the female, her masculine independence and strength wedded to thoroughly feminine grace of form and manner; may be said to give them both, through their double nature, command of life in all its phases, and a certain freemasonry of the secrets of the two sexes which may well favour their function as reconcilers and interpreters. Certainly it is remarkable that some of the world's greatest leaders and artists have been dowered either wholly or in part with the Uranian temperament—as in the cases of Michel Angelo, Shakespeare, Marlowe, Alexander the Great, Julius Cæsar, or, among women, Christine of Sweden, Sappho the poetess, and others.

III

THE HOMOGENIC ATTACHMENT

In its various forms, so far as we know them, Love seems always to have a deep significance and a most practical importance to us little mortals. In one form, as the mere semi-conscious Sex-love, which runs through creation and is common to the lowest animals and plants, it appears as a kind of organic basis for the unity of all creatures; in another, as the love of the mother for her offspring— which may also be termed a passion—it seems to pledge itself to the care and guardianship of the future race; in another, as the marriage of man and woman, it becomes the very foundation of human society. And so we can hardly believe that in its homogenic form, with which we are here concerned, it has not also a deep significance, and social uses and functions which will become clearer to us, the more we study it.

To some perhaps it may appear a little strained to place this last-mentioned form of attachment on a level of importance with the others, and such persons may be inclined to deny to the homogenic[12] or homosexual love that intense, that penetrating, and at times overmastering character which would entitle it to rank as a great human passion. But in truth this view, when entertained, arises from a want of acquaintance with the actual facts; and it may not be amiss here, in the briefest possible way, to indicate what the world's History, Literature, and Art has to say to us on this aspect of the subject, before going on to further considerations. Certainly, if the confronting of danger and the endurance of pain and distress for the sake of the loved one, if sacrifice, unswerving devotion and life-long union, constitute proofs of the reality and intensity (and let us say healthiness) of an affection, then these

---

[12] [Note: "Homosexual," generally used in scientific works is of course a bastard word. "Homogenic" has been suggested, as being from two roots, both Greek, i.e., "homos," same, and "genos," sex.]

proofs have been given in numberless cases of such attachment, not only as existing between men, but as between women, since the world began. The records of chivalric love, the feats of enamoured knights for their ladies' sakes, the stories of Hero and Leander, etc., are easily paralleled, if not surpassed, by the stories of the Greek comrades-in-arms and tyrannicides—of Cratinus and Aristodemus, who offered themselves together as a voluntary sacrifice for the purification of Athens; of Chariton and Melanippus, [13]who attempted to assassinate Phalaris, the tyrant of Agrigentum; or of Cleomachus who in like manner, in a battle between the Chalkidians and Eretrians, being entreated to charge the latter, "asked the youth he loved, who was standing by, whether he would be a spectator of the fight; and when he said he would, and affectionately kissed Cleomachus and put his helmet on his head, Cleomachus with a proud joy placed himself in the front of the bravest of the Thessalians and charged the enemy's cavalry with such impetuosity that he threw them into disorder and routed them; and the Eretrian cavalry fleeing in consequence, the Chalkidians won a splendid victory." [14]The annals of all nations contain similar records—though probably among none has the ideal of this love been quite so enthusiastic and heroic as among the post-Homeric Greeks. It is well known that among the Polynesian Islanders—for the most part a very gentle and affectionate people, probably inheriting the traditions of a higher culture than they now possess—the most romantic male friendships are (or were) in vogue. Says Herman Melville in "Omoo" (chap. 39), "The really curious way in which all Polynesians are in the habit of making bosom friends is deserving of remark. . . . In the annals of the island (Tahiti) are examples of extravagant friendships, unsurpassed by the story of Damon and Pythias—in truth much more wonderful; for notwithstanding the devotion—even of life in some cases— to which they led, they were frequently entertained at first sight for some stranger from another island." So thoroughly

---

[13] [Note: "Athenæus" xiii., ch. 78.]

[14] [Note: See Plutarch's "Eroticus," § xvii.]

recognised indeed were these unions that Melville explains (in "Typee," chap. 18) that if two men of hostile tribes or islands became thus pledged to each other, then each could pass through the enemy's territory without fear of molestation or injury; and the passionate nature of these attachments is indicated by the following passage from "Omoo":—"Though little inclined to jealousy in ordinary love-matters, the Tahitian will hear of no rivals in his friendship."

Even among savage races lower down than these in the scale of evolution, and who are generally accused of being governed in their love-relations only by the most animal desires, we find a genuine sentiment of comradeship beginning to assert itself—as among the Balonda [15]and other African tribes, where regular ceremonies of the betrothal of comrades take place, by the transfusion of a few drops of blood into each other's drinking- bowls, by the exchange of names, [16]and the mutual gift of their most precious possessions; but unfortunately, owing to the obtuseness of current European opinion on this subject, these and other such customs have been but little investigated and have by no means received the attention that they ought.

When we turn to the poetic and literary utterances of the more civilised nations on this subject we cannot but be struck by the range and intensity of the emotions expressed—from the beautiful threnody of David over his friend whose love was passing the love of women, through the vast panorama of the Homeric Iliad, of which the heroic friendship of Achilles and his dear Patroclus forms really the basic theme, down to the works of the great Greek age—the splendid odes of Pindar burning with clear fire of passion, the lofty elegies of Theognis, full of wise precepts to his beloved Kurnus, the sweet pastorals of Theocritus, the passionate lyrics of Sappho, or the more sensual raptures of Anacreon. Some of the dramas of Æschylus and Sophocles—as the "Myrmidones" of the former and the

---

[15] [Note: See "Natural History of Man," by J. G. Wood. Vol: "Africa," p. 419.]

[16] [Note: See also Livingstone's "Expedition to the Zambesi" (Murray, 1865) p. 148.]

"Lovers of Achilles" of the latter—appear to have had this subject for their motive; [17]and many of the prose-poem dialogues of Plato were certainly inspired by it.

Then coming to the literature of the Roman age, whose materialistic spirit could only with difficulty seize the finer inspiration of the homogenic love, and which in such writers as Catullus and Martial could only for the most part give expression to its grosser side, we still find in Vergil a noble and notable instance. His second Eclogue bears the marks of a genuine passion; and, according to some, [18]he there under the name of Alexis immortalises his own love for the youthful Alexander. Nor is it possible to pass over in this connection the great mass of Persian literature, and the poets Sadi, Hafiz, Jami, and many others, whose names and works are for all time, and whose marvellous love-songs ("Bitter and sweet is the parting kiss on the lips of a friend") are to a large extent, if not mostly, addressed to those of their own sex. [19]

Of the mediæval period in Europe we have of course but few literary monuments. Towards its close we come upon the interesting story of Amis and Amile (thirteenth century), unearthed by Mr. W. Pater from the Bibliotheca Elzeviriana. [20]Though there is historic evidence of the prevalence of the passion we may say of this period that its IDEAL was undoubtedly rather the chivalric love than the love of comrades. But with the Renaissance in Italy and the Elizabethan period in England the latter once more comes to evidence in a burst of poetic utterance, [21]which culminates perhaps in the magnificent sonnets of Michel Angelo and of Shakespeare; of Michel Angelo whose pure beauty of

[17] [Note: Though these two plays, except for some quotations, are lost.]

[18] [Note: Mantegazza and Lombroso. See Albert Moll, "Conträre Sexualempfindung," 2nd ed., p. 36.]

[19] [Note: Though in translation this fact is often by pious fraudulence disguised.]

[20] [Note: W. Pater's "Renaissance," pp. 8-16.]

[21] [Note: Among PROSE writers of this period, Montaigne, whose treatment of the subject is enthusiastic and unequivocal, should not be overlooked. See Hazlitt's "Montaigne," ch. xxvii.]

expression lifts the enthusiasm into the highest region as the direct perception of the divine in mortal form; [22]and of Shakespeare—whose passionate words and amorous spirituality of friendship have for long enough been a perplexity to hidebound commentators. Thence through minor writers (not overlooking Winckelmann [23] in Germany) we pass to quite modern times—in which, notwithstanding the fact that the passion has been much misunderstood and misinterpreted, two names stand conspicuously forth—those of Tennyson, whose "In Memoriam" is perhaps his finest work, and of Walt Whitman, the enthusiasm of whose poems on Comradeship is only paralleled by the devotedness of his labours for his wounded brothers in the American Civil War.

---

[22] [Note: I may be excused for quoting here the sonnet No. 54, from J. A. Symonds' translation of the sonnets of Michel Angelo:—

"From thy fair face I learn, O my loved lord,
That which no mortal tongue can rightly say:
The soul, imprisoned in her house of clay,
Holpen by thee to God hath often soared:
And though the vulgar, vain, malignant horde
Attribute what their grosser wills obey,
Yet shall this fervent homage that I pay,
This love, this faith, pure joys for us afford.
Lo, all the lovely things we find on earth,
Resemble for the soul that rightly sees,
That source of bliss divine which gave us birth:
Nor have we first-fruits or remembrances
Of heaven elsewhere. Thus, loving loyally,
I rise to God, and make death sweet by thee."

The labours of von Scheffler, followed by J. A. Symonds, have now pretty conclusively established the pious frauds of the nephew, and the fact that the love-poems of the elder Michel Angelo were, for the most part, written to male friends.]

[23] [Note: See an interesting paper in W. Pater's "Renaissance."]

It will be noticed that here we have some of the very greatest names in all literature concerned; and that their utterances on this subject equal if they do not surpass, in beauty, intensity and humanity of sentiment, whatever has been written in praise of the other more ordinarily recognised love.

And when again we turn to the records of Art, and compare the way in which man's sense of Love and Beauty has expressed itself in the portrayal of the male form and the female form respectively, we find exactly the same thing. The whole vista of Greek statuary shows the male passion of beauty in high degree. Yet though the statues of men and youths (by men sculptors) preponderate probably considerably, both in actual number and in devotedness of execution, over the statues of female figures, it is, as J. A. Symonds says in his "Life of Michel Angelo," remarkable that in all the range of the former there are hardly two or three that show a base or licentious expression, such as is not so very uncommon in the female statues. Knowing as we do the strength of the male physical passion in the life of the Greeks, this one fact speaks strongly for the sense of proportion which must have characterised this passion—at any rate in the most productive age of their Art.

In the case of Michel Angelo we have an artist who with brush and chisel portrayed literally thousands of human forms; but with this peculiarity, that while scores and scores of his male figures are obviously suffused and inspired by a romantic sentiment, there is hardly one of his female figures that is so,— the latter being mostly representative of woman in her part as mother, or sufferer, or prophetess or poetess, or in old age, or in any aspect of strength or tenderness, except that which associates itself especially with romantic love. Yet the cleanliness and dignity of Michel Angelo's male figures are incontestable, and bear striking witness to that nobility of the sentiment in him, which we have already seen illustrated in his sonnets. [24]This brief sketch may suffice to give the reader some

---

[24] [Note: For a fuller collection of instances of this Friendship-love in the history of the world, see "Ioläus: an Anthology," by E. Carpenter (George Allen, London, 1902).

idea of the place and position in the world of the particular sentiment which we are discussing; nor can it fail to impress him—if any reference is made to the authorities quoted—with a sense of the dignity and solidity of the sentiment, at any rate as handled by some of the world's greatest men. At the same time it would be affectation to ignore the fact that side by side with this view of the subject there has been another current of opinion leading people— especially in quite modern times in Europe—to look upon attachments of the kind in question with much suspicion and disfavour.[25] And it may be necessary here to say a few words on this latter view.

The origin of it is not far to seek. Those who have no great gift themselves for this kind of friendship—who are not in the inner circle of it, so to speak, and do not understand or appreciate its deep emotional and romantic character, have nevertheless heard of certain corruptions and excesses; for these latter leap to publicity. They have heard of the debaucheries of a Nero or a Tiberius; they have noted the scandals of the Police Courts; they have had some experience perhaps of abuses which may be found in Public Schools or Barracks; and they (not unnaturally) infer that these things, these excesses and sensualities, are the motive of comrade-attachments, and the object for which they exist; nor do they easily recognise any more profound and intimate bond. To such people physical intimacies of ANY kind (at any rate between males) seem inexcusable. There is no distinction in their minds between the simplest or most naive expression of feeling and the gravest abuse of human rights and decency; there is no distinction between a genuine heart-attachment and a mere carnal curiosity. They see certain evils that occur or have occurred, and they think, perfectly candidly, that any measures are justifiable to prevent such things recurring. But they do not

---

Also "Lieblingminne und Freundesliebe in der Weltliteratur," by Elisar von Kupffer (Adolf Brand, Berlin, 1900).]

[25] [Note: As in the case, for instance, of Tennyson's "In Memoriam," for which the poet was soundly rated by the Times at the time of its publication.]

see the interior love-feeling which when it exists does legitimately demand SOME expression. Such folk, in fact, not having the key in themselves to the real situation, hastily assume that the homogenic attachment has no other motive than, or is simply a veil and a cover for, sensuality—and suspect or condemn it accordingly.

Thus arises the curious discrepancy of people's views on this important subject—a discrepancy depending on the side from which they approach it.

On the one hand we have anathemas and execrations, on the other we have the lofty enthusiasm of a man like Plato— one of the leaders of the world's thought for all time—who puts, for example, into the mouth of Phædrus (in the "Symposium") such a passage as this:[26] "I know not any greater blessing to a young man beginning life than a virtuous lover, or to the lover than a beloved youth. For the principle which ought to be the guide of men who would nobly live—that principle, I say, neither kindred, nor honour, nor wealth, nor any other motive is able to implant so well as love. Of what am I speaking? Of the sense of honour and dishonour, without which neither states nor individuals ever do any good or great work. . . . For what lover would not choose rather to be seen of all mankind than by his beloved, either when abandoning his post or throwing away his arms? He would be ready to die a thousand deaths rather than endure this. Or who would desert his beloved or fail him in the hour of danger? The veriest coward would become an inspired hero, equal to the bravest, at such a time; love would inspire him. That courage which, as Homer says, the god breathes into the soul of heroes, love of his own nature inspires into the lover." Or again in the "Phædrus" Plato makes Socrates say[27]: "In like manner the followers of Apollo and of every other god, walking in the ways of their god, seek a love who is to be like their god, and when they have found him, they themselves imitate their god, and persuade their love to do the same, and bring him into harmony with the form and ways of the god as far as they can;

---

[26] [Note: Jowett's "Plato," 2nd ed., vol. ii., p. 30.]
[27] [Note: Jowett, vol. ii., p. 130.]

for they have no feelings of envy or jealousy towards their beloved, but they do their utmost to create in him the greatest likeness of themselves and the god whom they honour. Thus fair and blissful to the beloved when he is taken, is the desire of the inspired lover, and the initiation of which I speak into the mysteries of true love, if their purpose is effected."

With these few preliminary remarks we may pass on to consider some recent scientific investigations of the matter in hand. In late times—that is, during the last thirty years or so—a group of scientific and capable men chiefly in Germany, France, and Italy, have made a special and more or less impartial study of it. Among these may be mentioned Dr. Albert Moll of Berlin; R. von Krafft- Ebing, one of the leading medical authorities of Vienna, whose book on "Sexual Psychopathy" has passed into its tenth edition; Dr. Paul Moreau ("Des Aberrations du sens génésique"); Cesare Lombroso, the author of various works on Anthropology; M. A. Raffalovich ("Uranisme et unisexualité"); Auguste Forel ("Die Sexuelle Frage"); Mantegazza; K. H. Ulrichs; and last but not least, Dr. Havelock Ellis, of whose great work on the Psychology of Sex the second volume is dedicated to the subject of "Sexual Inversion."[28] The result of these investigations has been that a very altered complexion has been given to the subject. For whereas at first it was easily assumed that the phenomena were of morbid character, and that the leaning of the love-sentiment towards one of the same sex was always associated with degeneracy or disease, it is very noticeable that step by step with the accumulation of reliable information this assumption has been abandoned. The point of view has changed; and the change has been most marked in the latest authors, such as A. Moll and Havelock Ellis.

It is not possible here to go into anything like a detailed account of the works of these various authors, their theories,

---

[28] [Note: One ought also to mention some later writers, like Dr. Magnus Hirschfeld and Dr. von Römer, whose work, though avowedly favourable to the Urning movement, is in a high degree scientific and reliable in character.]

and the immense number of interesting cases and observations which they have contributed; but some of the general conclusions which flow from their researches may be pointed out. In the first place their labours have established the fact, known hitherto only to individuals, that SEXUAL INVERSION—that is the leaning of desire to one of the same sex—is in a vast number of cases quite instinctive and congenital, mentally and physically, and therefore twined in the very roots of individual life and practically ineradicable. To Men or Women thus affected with an innate homosexual bias, Ulrichs gave the name of Urning, [29]since pretty widely accepted by scientists. Some details with regard to "Urnings," I have given in the preceding paper, but it should be said here that too much emphasis cannot be laid on the distinction between these born lovers of their own kind, and that class of persons, with whom they are so often confused, who out of mere carnal curiosity or extravagance of desire, or from the dearth of opportunities for a more normal satisfaction (as in schools, barracks, etc.) adopt some homosexual practices. It is the latter class who become chiefly prominent in the public eye, and who excite, naturally enough, public reprobation. In their case the attraction is felt, by themselves and all concerned, to be merely sensual and morbid. In the case of the others, however, the feeling is, as said, so deeply rooted and twined with the mental and emotional life that the person concerned has difficulty in imagining himself affected otherwise than he is; and to him at least his love appears healthy and natural, and indeed a necessary part of his individuality.

In the second place it has become clear that the number of individuals affected with "sexual inversion" in some degree or other is very great—much greater than is generally supposed to be the case. It is however very difficult or perhaps impossible to arrive at satisfactory figures on the subject,[30] for the simple reasons that the proportions vary so greatly among different peoples and even in different sections of society and in

---

[29] [Note: From Uranos—see, for derivation, p. 20, supra—also Plato's "Symposium," speech of Pausanias.]

[30] [Note: See, for estimates, Appendix,]

32

different localities, and because of course there are all possible grades of sexual inversion to deal with, from that in which the instinct is QUITE EXCLUSIVELY directed towards the same sex, to the other extreme in which it is normally towards the opposite sex but capable, occasionally and under exceptional attractions, of inversion towards its own—this last condition being probably among some peoples very widespread, if not universal.

In the third place, by the tabulation and comparison of a great number of cases and "confessions," it has become pretty well established that the individuals affected with inversion in marked degree do not after all differ from the rest of mankind, or womankind, in any other physical or mental particular which can be distinctly indicated.[31] No congenital association with any particular physical conformation or malformation has yet been discovered; nor with any distinct disease of body or mind. Nor does it appear that persons of this class are usually of a gross or specially low type, but if anything rather the opposite—being mostly of refined, sensitive nature and including, as Krafft-Ebing points out ("Psychopathia Sexualis," seventh ed., p. 227) a great number "highly gifted in the fine arts, especially music and poetry"; and, as Mantegazza says, [32]many persons of high literary and social distinction. It is true that Krafft-Ebing insists on the generally strong sexual equipment of this class of persons (among men), but he hastens to say that their emotional love is also "enthusiastic and exalted," [33]and that, while bodily congress is desired, the special act with which they are vulgarly credited is in most cases repugnant to them. [34]

The only distinct characteristic which the scientific writers claim to have established is a marked tendency to nervous development in the subject, not infrequently associated with nervous maladies; but— as I shall presently have occasion to

---

[31] [Note: Though there is no doubt a general TENDENCY towards femininity of type in the male Urning, and towards masculinity in the female.]

[32] [Note: "Gli amori degli uomini."]

[33] [Note: "Psychopathia Sexualis," 7th ed., p. 227.]

[34] [Note: Ibid, pp. 229 and 258. See Appendix, p. 160.]

show—there is reason to think that the validity even of this characteristic has been exaggerated.

Taking the general case of men with a marked exclusive preference for persons of their own sex, Krafft-Ebing says ("P.S." p. 256): "The sexual life of these Homosexuals is mutatis mutandis just the same as in the case of normal sex-love . . . The Urning loves, deifies his male beloved one, exactly as the woman-wooing man does HIS beloved. For him, he is capable of the greatest sacrifice, experiences the torments of unhappy, often unrequited, love, of faithlessness on his beloved's part, of jealousy, and so forth. His attention is enchained only by the male form . . . The sight of feminine charms is indifferent to him, if not repugnant." Then he goes on to say that many such men, notwithstanding their actual aversion to intercourse with the female, do ultimately marry—either from ethical, as sometimes happens, or from social considerations. But very remarkable—as illustrating the depth and tenacity of the homogenic instinct[35]—and pathetic too, are the records that he gives of these cases; for in many of them a real friendship and regard between the married pair was still of no avail to overcome the distaste on the part of one to sexual intercourse with the other, or to prevent the experience of actual physical distress after such intercourse, or to check the continual flow of affection to some third person of the same sex; and thus unwillingly, so to speak, this bias remained a cause of suffering to the end.

I have said that at the outset it was assumed that the Homogenic emotion was morbid in itself, and probably always associated with distinct disease, either physical or mental, but that the progress of the inquiry has served more and more to dissipate this view; and that it is noticeable that the latest of the purely scientific authorities are the least disposed to insist upon the theory of morbidity. It is true that Krafft-Ebing clings to the opinion that there is generally some NEUROSIS, or

---

[35] [Note: "How deep congenital sex- inversion roots may be gathered from the fact that the pleasure- dream of the male Urning has to do with male persons, and of the female with females."—Krafft-Ebing, "P.S.," 7th ed., p. 228.]

degeneration of a nerve-centre, or INHERITED TENDENCY IN THAT DIRECTION, associated with the instinct; see p. 190 (seventh ed.), also p. 227, where he speaks, rather vaguely, of "an hereditary neuropathic or psychopathic tendency"— neuro(psycho)pathische Belastung. But it is an obvious criticism on this that there are few people in modern life, perhaps none, who could be pronounced absolutely free from such a Belastung! And whether the Dorian Greeks or the Polynesian Islanders or the Albanian mountaineers, or any of the other notably hardy races among whom this affection has been developed, were particularly troubled by nervous degeneration we may well doubt!

As to Moll, though he speaks [36] of the instinct as morbid (feeling perhaps in duty bound to do so), it is very noticeable that he abandons the ground of its association with other morbid symptoms—as this association, he says, is by no means always to be observed; and is fain to rest his judgment on the dictum that the mere failure of the sexual instinct to propagate the species is itself pathological—a dictum which in its turn obviously springs from that pre-judgment of scientists that generation is the sole object of love,[37] and which if pressed would involve the good doctor in awkward dilemmas, as for instance that every worker-bee is a pathological specimen.

Finally we find that Havelock Ellis, one of the latest writers of weight on this subject, in chapter vi. of his "Sexual Inversion," combats the idea that this temperament is necessarily morbid; and suggests that the tendency should rather be called an anomaly than a disease. He says (2nd edition, p. 186) [38]"Thus in sexual inversion we have what may fairly be called a 'sport' or variation, one of those organic aberrations which we see throughout living nature in plants and in animals." [39]

---

[36] [Note: "Conträre Sexualempfindung," 2nd ed., p. 269.]

[37] [Note: See "Love's Coming-of-Age," p. 22.]

[38] [Note: Pub.: F. A. Davis, Philadelphia, 1901.]

[39] [Note: Otto Weininger even goes further, and regards the temperament as a natural intermediate form ("Sex and Character," ch. iv.) See also Appendix, infra, p. 169.]

With regard to the nerve-degeneration theory, while it may be allowed that sexual inversion is not uncommonly found in connection with the specially nervous temperament, it must be remembered that its occasional association with nervous troubles or disease is quite another matter; since such troubles ought perhaps to be looked upon as the results rather than the causes of the inversion. It is difficult of course for outsiders not personally experienced in the matter to realise the great strain and tension of nerves under which those persons grow up from boyhood to manhood— or from girl to womanhood—who find their deepest and strongest instincts under the ban of the society around them; who before they clearly understand the drift of their own natures discover that they are somehow cut off from the sympathy and understanding of those nearest to them; and who know that they can never give expression to their tenderest yearnings of affection without exposing themselves to the possible charge of actions stigmatised as odious crimes.[40] That such a strain, acting on one who is perhaps already of a nervous temperament, should tend to cause nervous prostration or even mental disturbance is of course obvious; and if such disturbances are really found to be commoner among homogenic lovers than among ordinary folk we have in these social causes probably a sufficient explanation of the fact.

Then again in this connexion it must never be forgotten that the medico-scientific enquirer is bound on the whole to meet with those cases that are of a morbid character, rather than with those that ARE healthy in their manifestation, since indeed it is the former that he lays himself out for. And since the field of his research is usually a great modern city, there is little wonder if disease colours his conclusions. In the case of

---

[40] [Note: "Though then before my own conscience I cannot reproach myself, and though I must certainly reject the judgment of the world about us, yet I suffer greatly. In very truth I have injured no one, and I hold my love in its nobler activity for just as holy as that of normally disposed men, but under the unhappy fate that allows us neither sufferance nor recognition I suffer often more than my life can bear."—Extract from a letter given by Krafft-Ebing.]

Dr. Moll, who carried out his researches largely under the guidance of the Berlin police (whose acquaintance with the subject would naturally be limited to its least satisfactory sides), the only marvel is that his verdict is so markedly favourable as it is. As Krafft-Ebing says in his own preface, "It is the sad privilege of Medicine, and especially of Psychiatry, to look always on the reverse side of life, on the weakness and wretchedness of man."

Having regard then to the direction in which science has been steadily moving in this matter, it is not difficult to see that the epithet "morbid" will probably before long be abandoned as descriptive of the homogenic bias—that is, of the general sentiment of love towards a person of the same sex. That there are excesses of the passion—cases, as in ordinary sex-love, where mere physical desire becomes a mania—we may freely admit; but as it would be unfair to judge of the purity of marriage by the evidence of the Divorce courts, so it would be monstrous to measure the truth and beauty of the attachment in question by those instances which stand most prominently perhaps in the eye of the modern public; and after all deductions there remains, we contend, the vast body of cases in which the manifestation of the instinct has on the whole the character of normality and healthfulness— sufficiently so in fact to constitute this A DISTINCT VARIETY OF THE SEXUAL PASSION. The question, of course, not being whether the instinct is CAPABLE of morbid and extravagant manifestation—for that can easily be proved of any instinct— but whether it is capable of a healthy and sane expression. And this, we think, it has abundantly shown itself to be.

Anyhow the work that Science has practically done has been to destroy the dogmatic attitude of the former current opinion from which it itself started, and to leave the whole subject freed from a great deal of misunderstanding, and much more open than before. If on the one hand its results have been chiefly of a negative character, and it admits that it does not understand the exact place and foundation of this attachment; on the other hand since it recognises the deeply beneficial influences of an intimate love- relation of the usual kind on those concerned, it also allows that there are some persons for whom these necessary reactions can only come from one of the same sex as themselves.

"Successful love," says Moll (p. 125) "exercises a helpful influence on the Urning. His mental and bodily condition improves, and capacity of work increases—just as it happens in the case of a normal youth with HIS love." And further on (p. 173) in a letter from a man of this kind occur these words:— "The passion is I suppose so powerful, just because one looks for everything in the loved man—Love, Friendship, Ideal, and Sense- satisfaction. . . . As it is at present I suffer the agonies of a deep unresponded passion, which wake me like a nightmare from sleep. And I am conscious of physical pain in the region of the heart." In such cases the love, in some degree physically expressed, of another person of the same sex, is allowed to be as much a necessity and a condition of healthy life and activity, as in more ordinary cases is the love of a person of the opposite sex.

If then the physical element which is sometimes present in the love of which we are speaking is a difficulty and a stumbling-block, it must be allowed that it is a difficulty that Nature confronts us with, and which cannot be disposed of by mere anathema and execration. The only theory—from K. H. Ulrichs to Havelock Ellis— which has at all held its ground in this matter, is that in congenital cases of sex-inversion there is a mixture of male and female elements in the same person; so that for instance in the same embryo the emotional and nervous regions may develop along feminine lines while the outer body and functions may determine themselves as distinctly masculine, or vice versa. Such cross- development may take place obviously in a great variety of ways, and thus possibly explain the remarkable varieties of the Uranian temperament; but in all such cases, strange as may be the problems thus arising, these problems are of Nature's own producing and can hardly be laid to the door of the individual who has literally to bear their cross. For such individuals expressions of feeling become natural, which to others seem out of place and uncalled for; and not only natural, but needful and inevitable. To deny to such people ALL expression of their emotion, is probably in the end to cause it to burst forth with the greater violence; and it may be suggested that our British code of manners, by forbidding the lighter marks of affection between youths and men, acts just contrary to its own purpose, and drives intimacies down into less open and unexceptionable channels.

With regard to this physical element it must also be remembered that since the homogenic love—whether between man and man, or between woman and woman—can from the nature of the case never find expression on the physical side so freely and completely as is the case with the ordinary love, it must tend rather more than the latter to run along EMOTIONAL channels, and to find its vent in sympathies of social life and companionship. If one studies carefully the expression of the Greek statues (see p. 9, supra) and the lesson of the Greek literature, one sees clearly that the IDEAL of Greek life was a very continent one: the trained male, the athlete, the man temperate and restrained, even chaste, for the sake of bettering his powers. It was round this conception that the Greeks kindled their finer emotions. And so of their love: a base and licentious indulgence was not in line with it. They may not have always kept to their ideal, but there it was. And I am inclined to think that the homogenic instinct (for the reasons given above) would in the long run tend to work itself out in this direction. And consonant with this is the fact that this passion in the past (as pointed out by J. Addington Symonds in his paper on "Dantesque and Platonic Ideals of Love"[41]) has, as a matter of fact, inspired such a vast amount of heroism and romance— only paralleled indeed by the loves of Chivalry, which of course, owing to their special character, were subject to a similar Transmutation.

In all these matters the popular opinion has probably been largely influenced by the arbitrary notion that the function of love is limited to child-breeding; and that any love not concerned in the propagation of the race must necessarily be of dubious character. And in enforcing this view, no doubt the Hebraic and Christian tradition has exercised a powerful

---

[41] [Note: See "In the Key of Blue," by J. A. Symonds (Elkin Mathews, 1893).]

influence—dating, as it almost certainly does, from far-back times when the multiplication of the tribe was one of the first duties of its members, and one of the first necessities of corporate life. [42]But nowadays when the need has swung round all the other way it is not unreasonable to suppose that a similar revolution will take place in people's views of the place and purpose of the non-child-bearing love. [43]

————

I have now said enough I think to show that though much in relation to the homogenic attachment is obscure, and though it may have its special pitfalls and temptations—making it quite necessary to guard against a too great latitude on the physical side; yet on its ethical and social sides it is pregnant with meaning and has received at various times in history abundant justification. It certainly does not seem impossible to suppose that as the ordinary love has a special function in the propagation of the race, so the other has its special function in social and heroic work, and in the generation—not of bodily children—but of those children of the mind, the philosophical conceptions and ideals which transform our lives and those of society. J. Addington Symonds, in his privately printed pamphlet, "A Problem in Greek Ethics" (now published in a German translation), [44]endeavours to reconstruct as it were the genesis of comrade-love among the Dorians in early Greek times. Thus:— "Without sufficiency of women, without the sanctities of established domestic life, inspired by the memories of Achilles and venerating their ancestor Herakles, the Dorian warriors had special opportunity for elevating comradeship to the rank of an enthusiasm. The incidents of emigration into a foreign country—perils of the sea, passages of rivers and mountains, assaults of fortresses and cities, landings on a hostile shore, night-vigils by the side of blazing beacons, foragings for food, picquet service in the front of watchful foes—involved adventures capable of shedding the lustre of

————

[42] [Note: See Appendix, pp. 162 and 163.]

[43] [Note: See also "Love's Coming-of-Age," 5th ed., pp. 173, 174.]

[44] [Note: See "Das Conträre Geschlechtsgefühl," by Havelock Ellis and J. A. Symonds (Leipzig, 1896).]

romance on friendship. These circumstances, by bringing the virtues of sympathy with the weak, tenderness for the beautiful, protection for the young, together with corresponding qualities of gratitude, self-devotion, and admiring attachment into play, may have tended to cement unions between man and man no less firm than that of marriage. On such connections a wise captain would have relied for giving strength to his battalions, and for keeping alive the flames of enterprise and daring." The author then goes on to suggest that though in such relations as those indicated the physical probably had some share, yet it did not at that time overbalance the emotional and spiritual elements, or lead to the corruption and effeminacy of a later age.

At Sparta the lover was called Eispnêlos, the inspirer, and the younger beloved Aïtes, the hearer. This alone would show the partly educational aspects in which comradeship was conceived; and a hundred passages from classic literature might be quoted to prove how deeply it had entered into the Greek mind that this love was the cradle of social chivalry and heroic life. Finally it seems to have been Plato's favourite doctrine that the relation if properly conducted led up to the disclosure of true philosophy in the mind, to the divine vision or mania, and to the remembrance or rekindling within the soul of all the forms of celestial beauty. He speaks of this kind of love as causing a "generation in the beautiful" [45]within the souls of the lovers. The image of the beloved one passing into the mind of the lover and upward through its deepest recesses reaches and unites itself to the essential forms of divine beauty there long hidden—the originals as it were of all creation—and stirring them to life excites a kind of generative descent of noble thoughts and impulses, which henceforward modify the whole cast of thought and life of the one so affected.

If there is any truth—even only a grain or two—in these speculations, it is easy to see that the love with which we are specially dealing is a very important factor in society, and that its neglect, or its repression, or its vulgar misapprehension, may be matters of considerable danger or damage to the common-

---

[45] [Note: "Symposium," Speech of Socrates.]

weal. It is easy to see that while on the one hand marriage is of indispensable importance to the State as providing the workshop as it were for the breeding and rearing of children, another form of union is almost equally indispensable to supply the basis for social activities of other kinds. Every one is conscious that without a close affectional tie of some kind his life is not complete, his powers are crippled, and his energies are inadequately spent. Yet it is not to be expected (though it may of course happen) that the man or woman who have dedicated themselves to each other and to family life should leave the care of their children and the work they have to do at home in order to perform social duties of a remote and less obvious, though may be more arduous, character. Nor is it to be expected that a man or woman single-handed, without the counsel of a helpmate in the hour of difficulty, or his or her love in the hour of need, should feel equal to these wider activities. If—to refer once more to classic story—the love of Harmodius had been for a wife and children at home, he would probably not have cared, and it would hardly have been his business, to slay the tyrant. And unless on the other hand each of the friends had had the love of his comrade to support him, the two could hardly have nerved themselves to this audacious and ever-memorable exploit. So it is difficult to believe that anything can supply the force and liberate the energies required for social and mental activities of the most necessary kind so well as a comrade-union which yet leaves the two lovers free from the responsibilities and impedimenta of family life.

For if the slaughter of tyrants is not the chief social duty now-a- days, we have with us hydra-headed monsters at least as numerous as the tyrants of old, and more difficult to deal with, and requiring no little courage to encounter. And beyond the extirpation of evils we have solid work waiting to be done in the patient and lifelong building up of new forms of society, new orders of thought, and new institutions of human solidarity—all of which in their genesis must meet with opposition, ridicule, hatred, and even violence. Such campaigns as these—though different in kind from those of the Dorian mountaineers described above—will call for equal hardihood and courage, and will stand in need of a comradeship as true and valiant. And it may indeed be doubted whether the higher heroic and spiritual life of a nation is ever quite possible without the sanction of this attachment in its institutions, adding a new range and scope to the possibilities of love. [46]

Walt Whitman, the inaugurator, it may almost be said, of a new world of democratic ideals and literature, and—as one of the best of our critics has remarked—the most Greek in spirit and in performance of modern writers, insists continually on this social function of "intense and loving comradeship, the personal and passionate attachment of man to man." "I will make," he says, "the most splendid race the sun ever shone upon, I will make divine magnetic lands. . . . I will make inseparable cities with their arms about each others' necks, by the love of comrades." And again, in "Democratic Vistas," "It is to the development, identification, and general prevalence of that fervid comradeship (the adhesive love at least rivalling the amative love hitherto possessing imaginative literature, if not going beyond it), that I look for the counterbalance and offset of materialistic and vulgar American Democracy, and for the spiritualisation thereof. . . . I say Democracy infers such loving comradeship, as its most inevitable twin or counterpart, without which it will be incomplete, in vain, and incapable of perpetuating itself."

Yet Whitman could not have spoken, as he did, with a kind of authority on this subject, if he had not been fully aware that through the masses of the people this attachment was already

---

[46] [Note: It is interesting in this connection to notice the extreme fervour, almost of romance, of the bond which often unites lovers of like sex over a long period of years, in an unfailing tenderness of treatment and consideration towards each other, equal to that shown in the most successful marriages. The love of many such men, says Moll (p. 119), "developed in youth lasts at times the whole life through. I know of such men, who had not seen their first love for years, even decades, and who yet on meeting showed the old fire of their first passion. In other cases, a close love- intimacy will last unbroken for many years."]

alive and working—though doubtless in a somewhat suppressed and un-self- conscious form—and if he had not had ample knowledge of its effects and influence in himself and others around him. Like all great artists he could but give form and light to that which already existed dim and inchoate in the heart of the people. To those who have dived at all below the surface in this direction it will be familiar enough that the homogenic passion ramifies widely through all modern society, and that among the masses of the people as among the classes, even below the stolid surface and reserve of British manners, letters pass and enduring attachments are formed, differing in no very obvious respect from those correspondences which persons of opposite sex knit with each other under similar circumstances; but that hitherto while this relation has occasionally, in its grosser forms and abuses, come into public notice through the police reports, etc., its more sane and spiritual manifestations—though really a moving force in the body politic—have remained unrecognised.

It is hardly needful in these days when social questions loom so large upon us to emphasise the importance of a bond which by the most passionate and lasting compulsion may draw members of the different classes together, and (as it often seems to do) none the less strongly because they are members of different classes. A moment's consideration must convince us that such a comradeship may, as Whitman says, have "deepest relations to general politics." It is noticeable, too, in this deepest relation to politics that the movement among women towards their own liberation and emancipation, which is taking place all over the civilised world, has been accompanied by a marked development of the homogenic passion among the female sex. It may be said that a certain strain in the relations between the opposite sexes which has come about owing to a growing consciousness among women that they have been oppressed and unfairly treated by men, and a growing unwillingness to ally themselves unequally in marriage—that this strain has caused the womenkind to draw more closely together and to cement alliances of their own. But whatever the cause may be, it is pretty certain that such comrade-alliances—and of quite devoted kind—are becoming increasingly common, and especially perhaps among the more cultured classes of women, who are working out the great cause of their sex's liberation; nor is it difficult to see the importance of such alliances in such a campaign. In the United States where the battle of women's independence is also being fought, the tendency mentioned is as strongly marked.

A few words may here be said about the legal aspect of this important question. It has to be remarked that the present state of the Law, both in Germany and Britain—arising as it does partly out of some of the misapprehensions above alluded to, and partly out of the sheer unwillingness of legislators to discuss the question—is really impracticable. While the Law rightly seeks to prevent acts of violence or public scandal, it may be argued that it is going beyond its province when it attempts to regulate the private and voluntary relations of adult persons to each other. The homogenic affection is a valuable social force, and in some cases a necessary element of noble human character—yet the Act of 1885 makes almost any familiarity in such cases the possible basis of a criminal charge. The Law has no doubt had substantial ground for previous statutes on this subject—dealing with a certain gross act; but in so severely condemning the least familiarity between male persons [47] we think it has gone too far. It has undertaken a censorship over private morals (entirely apart from social results) which is beyond its province, and which— even if it were its province—it could not possibly fulfil;[48] it has opened wider than ever before the door to a real, most serious social evil and crime—that of blackmailing; and it has thrown a shadow over even the simplest and most ordinary expressions of an attachment which may, as we have seen, be of great value in the national life.

That the homosexual feeling, like the heterosexual, may lead to public abuses of liberty and decency; that it needs a

---

[47] [Note: Though, inconsistently enough, making no mention of females.]

[48] [Note: Dr. Moll maintains (2nd ed., pp. 314, 315) that if familiarities between those of the same sex are made illegal, as immoral, self- abuse ought much more to be so made.]

strict self- control; and that much teaching and instruction on the subject is needed; we of course do not deny. But as, in the case of persons of opposite sex, the law limits itself on the whole to a maintenance of public order, the protection of the weak from violence and insult,[49] and of the young from their inexperience; so we think it should be here. The much-needed teaching and the true morality on the subject must be given—as it can only be given—by the spread of proper education and ideas, and not by the clumsy bludgeon of the statute-book. [50]

Having thus shown the importance of the homogenic or comrade-attachment, in some form, in national life, it would seem high time now that the modern peoples should recognise this in their institutions, and endeavour at least in their public opinion and systems of education to understand this factor and give it its proper place. The undoubted evils which exist in relation to it, for instance in our public schools as well as in our public life, owe their existence largely to the fact that the whole subject is left in the gutter so to speak—in darkness and concealment. No one offers a clue of better things, nor to point a way out of the wilderness; and by this very non-recognition the passion is perverted into its least satisfactory channels. All love, one would say, must have its responsibilities, else it is liable to degenerate, and to dissipate itself in mere sentiment or sensuality. The normal marriage between man and woman leads up to the foundation of the household and the family; the love between parents and children implies duties and cares on both sides. The homogenic attachment, left unrecognised, easily loses some of its best quality and becomes an ephemeral or corrupt thing. Yet, as we have seen, and as I am pointing out in the following chapter, it may, when occurring between an elder

---

[49] [Note: Though it is doubtful whether the marriage-laws even do this.]

[50] [Note: In France, since the adoption of the Code Napoleon, sexual inversion is tolerated under the same restrictions as normal sexuality; and according to Carlier, formerly Chief of the French Police, Paris is not more depraved in this matter than London. Italy in 1889 also adopted the principles of the Code Napoleon on this point. For further considerations with regard to the Law, see Appendix, pp. 164 and 165.]

and younger, prove to be an immense educational force; while, as between equals, it may be turned to social and heroic uses, such as can hardly be demanded or expected from the ordinary marriage. It would seem high time, I say, that public opinion should recognise these facts; and so give to this attachment the sanction and dignity which arise from public recognition, as well as the definite form and outline which would flow from the existence of an accepted ideal or standard in the matter. It is often said how necessary for the morality of the ordinary marriage is some public recognition of the relation, and some accepted standard of conduct in it. May not, to a lesser degree, something of the same kind (as suggested in the next chapter) be true of the homogenic attachment? It has had its place as a recognised and guarded institution in the elder and more primitive societies; and it seems quite probable that a similar place will be accorded to it in the societies of the future.

IV

AFFECTION IN EDUCATION

The place of Affection, and the need of it, as an educative force in school-life, is a subject which is beginning to attract a good deal of attention. Hitherto Education has been concentred on intellectual (and physical) development; but the affections have been left to take care of themselves. Now it is beginning to be seen that the affections have an immense deal to say in the building up of the brain and the body. Their evolution and organisation in some degree is probably going to become an important part of school management.

School friendships of course exist; and almost every one remembers that they filled a large place in the outlook of his early years; but he remembers, too, that they were not recognised in any way, and that in consequence the main part of their force and value was wasted. Yet it is evident that the first unfolding of a strong attachment in boyhood or girlhood must have a profound influence; while if it occurs between an elder and a younger school- mate, or—as sometimes happens—between the young thing and its teacher, its importance in the educational sense can hardly be overrated.

That such feelings sometimes take quite intense and romantic forms few will deny. I have before me a letter, in which the author, speaking of an attachment he experienced when a boy of sixteen for a youth somewhat older than himself, says:—

"I would have died for him ten times over. My devices and plannings to meet him (to come across him casually, as it were) were those of a lad for his sweetheart, and when I saw him my heart beat so violently that it caught my breath, and I could not speak. We met in ——, and for the weeks that he stayed there I thought of nothing else—thought of him night and day—and when he returned to London I used to write him weekly letters, veritable love-letters of many sheets in length. Yet I never felt one particle of jealousy, though our friendship lasted for some years. The passion, violent and extravagant as it was, I believe to have been perfectly free from sex-feeling and perfectly wholesome and good for me. It distinctly contributed to my growth. Looking back upon it and analysing it as well as I can, I seem to see as the chief element in it an escape from the extremely narrow Puritanism in which I was reared, into a large sunny ingenuous nature which knew nothing at all of the bondage of which I was beginning to be acutely conscious."

Shelley in his fragmentary "Essay on Friendship" speaks in the most glowing terms of an attachment he formed at school, and so does Leigh Hunt in his "Autobiography." Says the latter:—

"If I had reaped no other benefit from Christ Hospital, the school would be ever dear to me from the recollection of the friendships I formed in it, and of the first heavenly taste it gave me of that most spiritual of the affections. . . . I shall never forget the impression it made on me. I loved my friend for his gentleness, his candour, his truth, his good repute, his freedom even from my own livelier manner, his calm and reasonable kindness. . . . I doubt whether he ever had a conception of a tithe of the regard and respect I entertained for him, and I smile to think of the perplexity (though he never showed it) which he probably felt sometimes at my enthusiastic expressions; for I thought him a kind of angel."

It is not necessary, however, to quote authorities on such a subject as this.[51] Any one who has had experience of schoolboys knows well enough that they are capable of forming these romantic and devoted attachments, and that their alliances are often of the kind especially referred to as having a bearing on education—i.e., between an elder and a younger. They are genuine attractions, free as a rule, and at their inception, from secondary motives. They are not formed by the elder one for any personal ends. More often, indeed, I think they are begun by the younger, who naively allows his admiration of the elder one to become visible. But they are absorbing and intense, and on either side their influence is deeply felt and long remembered.

---

[51] [Note: For further instances, see Appendix,]

That such attachments MAY be of the very greatest value is self- evident. The younger boy looks on the other as a hero, loves to be with him, thrills with pleasure at his words of praise or kindness, imitates, and makes him his pattern and standard, learns exercises and games, contracts habits, or picks up information from him. The elder one, touched, becomes protector and helper; the unselfish side of his nature is drawn out, and he develops a real affection and tenderness towards the younger. He takes all sorts of trouble to initiate his protégé in field sports or studies; is proud of the latter's success; and leads him on perhaps later to share his own ideals of life and thought and work.

Sometimes the alliance will begin, in a corresponding way, from the side of the elder boy. Sometimes, as said, between a boy and a master such an attachment, or the germ of it, is found; and indeed it is difficult to say what gulf, or difference of age, or culture, or class in society, is so great that affection of this kind will not on occasion overpass it. I have by me a letter which was written by a boy of eleven or twelve to a young man of twenty-four or twenty-five. The boy was rather a wild, "naughty" boy, and had given his parents (working-class folk) a good deal of trouble. He attended, however, some sort of night-school or evening class and there conceived the strongest affection (evidenced by this letter) for his teacher, the young man in question, quite spontaneously, and without any attempt on the part of the latter to elicit it; and (which was equally important) without any attempt on his part to deny it. The result was most favourable; the one force which could really reach the boy had, as it were, been found; and he developed rapidly and well.

The following extract is from a letter written by an elderly man who has had large experience as a teacher. He says—

"It has always seemed to me that the rapport that exists between two human beings, whether of the same or of different sexes, is a force not sufficiently recognised, and capable of producing great results. Plato fully understood its importance, and aimed at giving what to his countrymen was more or less sensual, a noble and exalted direction. . . . As one who has had much to do in instructing boys and starting them in life, I am convinced that the great secret of being a good teacher consists in the possibility of that rapport; not only of a merely intellectual nature, but involving a certain physical clement, a personal affection, almost indescribable, that grows up between pupil and teacher, and through which thoughts are shared and an influence created that could exist in no other way."

And it must be evident to every one that to the expanding mind of a small boy to have a relation of real affection with some sensible and helpful elder of his own sex must be a priceless boon. At that age love to the other sex has hardly declared itself, and indeed is not exactly what is wanted. The unformed mind requires an ideal of itself, as it were, to which it can cling or towards which it can grow. Yet it is equally evident that the relation and the success of it, will depend immensely on the character of the elder one, on the self-restraint and tenderness of which he is capable, and on the ideal of life which he has in his mind. That, possibly, is the reason why Greek custom, at least in the early days of Hellas, not only recognised friendships between elder and younger youths as a national institution of great importance, but laid down very distinct laws or rules concerning the conduct of them, so as to be a guide and a help to the elder in what was acknowledged to be a position of responsibility.

In Crete, for instance, [52]the friendship was entered into in quite a formal and public way, with the understanding and consent of relatives; the position of the elder was clearly defined, and it became his business to train and exercise the younger in skill of arms, the chase, etc.; while the latter could obtain redress at law if the elder subjected him to insult or injury of any kind. At the end of a certain period of probation, if the younger desired it he could leave his comrade; if not, he became his squire or henchman—the elder being bound to furnish his military equipments—and they fought thenceforward side by side in battle, "inspired with double valour, according to the notions of the Cretans, by the gods of

---

[52] [Note: See Müller's "History and Antiquities of the Doric Race."]

war and love." [53]Similar customs prevailed in Sparta, and, in a less defined way, in other Greek states; as, indeed, they have prevailed among many semi- barbaric races on the threshold of civilisation.

When, however, we turn to modern life and the actual situation, as for instance in the public schools of to-day, it may well be objected that we find very little of the suggested ideal, but rather an appalling descent into the most uninspiring conditions. So far from friendship being an institution whose value is recognised and understood, it is at best scantily acknowledged, and is often actually discountenanced and misunderstood. And though attachments such as we have portrayed exist, they exist underground, as it were, at their peril, and half-stifled in an atmosphere which can only be described as that of the gutter. Somehow the disease of premature sexuality seems to have got possession of our centres of education; wretched practices and habits abound, and (what is perhaps their worst feature) cloud and degrade the boys' conception of what true love or friendship may be.

To those who are familiar with large public schools the state of affairs does not need describing. A friend (who has placed some notes at my disposal) says that in his time a certain well-known public school was a mass of uncleanness, incontinence, and dirty conversation, while at the same time a great deal of genuine affection, even to heroism, was shown among the boys in their relations with one another. But "all these things were treated by masters and boys alike as more or less unholy, with the result that they were either sought after or flung aside according to the sexual or emotional instinct of the boy. No attempt was made at discrimination. A kiss was by comparison as unclean as the act of fellatio, and no one had any gauge or principle whatever on which to guide the cravings of boyhood." The writer then goes into details which it is not necessary to reproduce here. He (and others) were initiated in the mysteries of sex by the dormitory servant; and the boys thus corrupted mishandled each other.

---

[53] [Note: Müller.]

Naturally in any such atmosphere as this the chances AGAINST the formation of a decent and healthy attachment are very large. If the elder youth happen to be given to sensuality he has here his opportunity; if on the other hand he is NOT given to it, the ideas current around probably have the effect of making him suspect his own affection, and he ends by smothering and disowning the best part of his nature. In both ways harm is done. The big boys in such places become either coarse and licentious or hard and self- righteous; the small boys, instead of being educated and strengthened by the elder ones, become effeminate little wretches, the favourites, the petted boys, and the "spoons" of the school. As time goes on the public opinion of the school ceases to believe in the possibility of a healthy friendship; the masters begin to presume (and not without reason) that all affection means sensual practices, and end by doing their best to discourage it.

Now this state of affairs is really desperate. There is no need to be puritanical, or to look upon the lapses of boyhood as unpardonable sins; indeed, it may be allowed, as far as that goes, that a little frivolity is better than hardness and self-righteousness; yet every one feels, and must feel, who knows anything about the matter, that the state of our schools is bad.

And it is so because, after all, purity (in the sense of continence) IS of the first importance to boyhood. To prolong the period of continence in a boy's life is to prolong the period of GROWTH. This is a simple physiological law, and a very obvious one; and whatever other things may be said in favour of purity, it remains perhaps the most weighty. To introduce sensual and sexual habits—and one of the worst of these is self-abuse—at an early age, is to arrest growth, both physical and mental.

And what is even more, it means to arrest the capacity for affection. I believe affection, attachment—whether to the one sex or the other—springs up normally in the youthful mind in a quite diffused, ideal, emotional form—a kind of longing and amazement as at something divine—with no definite thought or distinct consciousness of sex in it. The sentiment expands and fills, as it were like a rising tide, every cranny of the emotional and moral nature; and the longer (of course within reasonable limits) its definite outlet towards sex is deferred, the longer does this period of emotional growth and development continue, and the greater is the refinement and breadth and strength of character resulting. All experience shows that a too early outlet towards sex cheapens and weakens affectional capacity.

Yet this early outlet it is which is the great trouble of our public schools. And it really does not seem unlikely that the peculiar character of the middle-class man of to-day, his undeveloped affectional nature and something of brutishness and woodenness, is largely due to the prevalent condition of the places of his education. The Greeks, with their wonderful instinct of fitness, seem to have perceived the right path in all this matter; and, while encouraging friendship, as we have seen, made a great point of modesty in early life—the guardians and teachers of every well-born boy being especially called upon to watch over the sobriety of his habits and manners.[54]

We have then in education generally, it seems to me (and whether of boys or of girls), two great currents to deal with, which cannot be ignored, and which certainly ought to be candidly recognized and given their right direction. One of these currents is that of friendship. The other is that of the young thing's natural curiosity about sex. The latter is of course, or should be, a perfectly legitimate interest. A boy at puberty naturally wants to know—and ought to know—what is taking place, and what the uses and functions of his body are. He does not go very deep into things; a small amount of information will probably satisfy him; but the curiosity is there, and it is pretty certain that the boy, if he is a boy of any sense or character, WILL in some shape or another get to satisfy it.

The process is really a MENTAL one. Desire—except in some abnormal cases—has not manifested itself strongly; and there is often, perhaps generally, an actual repugnance at first to anything like sexual practices; but the wish for information

---

[54] [Note: Cf. the incident at the end of Plato's "Lysis," when the tutors of Lysis and Menexenus come in and send the youths home.]

54

exists and is, I say, legitimate enough.[55] In almost all human societies except, curiously, the modern nations, there have been institutions for the initiation of the youth of either sex into these matters, and these initiations have generally been associated, in the opening blossom of the young mind, with inculcation of the ideals of manhood and womanhood, courage, hardihood, and the duties of the citizen or the soldier.[56]

But what does the modern school do? It shuts a trap-door down on the whole matter. There is a hush; a grim silence. Legitimate curiosity soon becomes illegitimate of its kind; and a furtive desire creeps in, where there was no desire before. The method of the gutter prevails. In the absence of any recognition of schoolboy needs, contraband information is smuggled from one to another; chaff and "smut" take the place of sensible and decent explanations; unhealthy practices follow; the sacredness of sex goes its way, never to return, and the school is filled with premature and morbid talk and thought about a subject which should, by rights, only just be rising over the mental horizon.

The meeting of these two currents, of ideal attachment and sexual desire, constitutes a rather critical period, even when it takes place in the normal way—i.e., later on, and at the matrimonial age. Under the most favourable conditions a certain conflict occurs in the mind at their first encounter. But in the modern school this conflict, precipitated far too soon, and accompanied by an artificial suppression of the nobler current and a premature hastening of the baser one, ends in simple disaster to the former. Masters wage war against incontinence, and are right to do so. But how do they wage it? As said, by grim silence and fury, by driving the abscess deeper, by covering the drain over, AND by confusing when it comes

---

[55] [Note: For a useful little manual on this subject, see "How We are Born," by Mrs. N. J. (Daniel, London). For a general argument in favour of sex-teaching see "The Training of the Young in Laws of Sex," by Canon Lyttelton, Headmaster of Eton College (Longmans).]
[56] [Note: See J. G. Wood's "Natural History of Man," vol. "Africa," p. 324 (the Bechuanas); also vol. "Australia," p. 75.]

before them—both in their own minds and those of the boys—a real attachment with that which they condemn.

Not long ago the head-master of a large public school coming suddenly out of his study chanced upon two boys embracing each other in the corridor. Possibly, and even probably, it was the simple and natural expression of an unsophisticated attachment. Certainly, it was nothing that in itself could be said to be either right or wrong. What did he do? He haled the two boys into his study, gave them a long lecture on the nefariousness of their conduct, with copious hints that he knew WHAT SUCH THINGS MEANT, and WHAT THEY LED TO, and ended by punishing both condignly. Could anything be more foolish? If their friendship was clean and natural, the master was only trying to make them feel that it was unclean and unnatural, and that a lovely and honourable thing was disgraceful; if the act was—which at least is improbable—a mere signal of lust—even then the best thing would have been to assume that it was honourable, and by talking to the boys, either together or separately, to try and inspire them with a better ideal; while if, between these positions, the master really thought the affection though honourable would lead to things undesirable, then, plainly, to punish the two was only to cement their love for each other, to give them a strong reason for concealing it, and to hasten its onward course. Yet every one knows that this is the KIND of way in which the subject is treated in schools. It is the method of despair. And masters (perhaps not unnaturally) finding that they have not the time which would be needed for personal dealing with each boy, nor the forces at their command by which they might hope to introduce new ideals of life and conduct into their little community, and feeling thus utterly unable to cope with the situation, allow themselves to drift into a policy of mere silence with regard to it, tempered by outbreaks of ungoverned and unreasoning severity.

I venture to think that school-masters will never successfully solve the difficulty until they boldly recognize the two needs in question, and proceed candidly to give them their proper satisfaction.

The need of information—the legitimate curiosity—of boys (and girls) must be met, (1) partly by classes on physiology, (2) partly by private talks and confidences between elder and younger, based on friendship. With regard to (1) classes of this kind are already, happily, being carried on at a few advanced schools, and with good results. And though such classes can only go rather generally into the facts of motherhood and generation they cannot fail, if well managed, to impress the young minds, and give them a far grander and more reverent conception of the matter than they usually gain.

But (2) although some rudimentary teaching on sex and lessons in physiology may be given in classes, it is obvious that further instruction and indeed any real help in the conduct of life and morals can only come through very close and tender confidences between the elder and the younger, such as exist where there is a strong friendship to begin with. It is obvious that effective help CAN only come in this way, and that this is the only way in which it is desirable that it should come. The elder friend in this case would, one might say, naturally be, and in many instances may be, the parent, mother or father—who ought certainly to be able to impress on the clinging child the sacredness of the relation. And it is much to be hoped that parents will see their way to take this part more freely in the future. But for some unexplained reason there is certainly often a gulf of reserve between the (British) parent and child; and the boy who is much at school comes more under the influence of his elder companions than his parents. If, therefore, boys and youths cannot be trusted and encouraged to form decent and loving friendships with each other, and with their elders or juniors—in which many delicate questions could be discussed and the tradition of sensible and manly conduct with regard to sex handed down—we are indeed in a bad plight and involved in a vicious circle from which escape seems difficult.

And so (we think) the need of attachment must also be met by full recognition of it, and the granting of it expression within all reasonable limits; by the dissemination of a good ideal of friendship and the enlistment of it on the side of manliness and temperance. Is it too much to hope that schools will in time recognise comradeship as a regular institution—considerably more important, say, than "fagging"—an institution having its definite place in the school life, in the games and in the studies, with its own duties, responsibilities, privileges, etc., and serving to ramify through the little community, hold it together, and inspire its members with the two qualities of heroism and tenderness, which together form the basis of all great character?

But here it must be said that if we are hoping for any great change in the conduct of our large boys' schools, the so-called public schools are not the places in which to look for it—or at any rate for its inception. In the first place these institutions are hampered by powerful traditions which naturally make them conservative; and in the second place their mere size and the number of boys make them difficult to deal with or to modify. The masters are overwhelmed with work; and the (necessary) division of so many boys into separate "houses" has this effect that a master who introduces a better tradition into his own house has always the prospect before him that his work will be effaced by the continual and perhaps contaminating contact with the boys from the other houses. No, it will be in smaller schools, say of from 50 to 100 boys, where the personal influence of the headmaster will be a real force reaching each boy, and where he will be really able to mould the tradition of the school, that we shall alone be able to look for an improved state of affairs.[57] No doubt the first steps in any reform of this

---

[57] [Note: With the rapid rise which is taking place, in scope and social status, of the state day- schools, it is probable that some change of opinion will take place with regard to the wisdom of sending young boys of ten to fourteen to upper-class boarding-schools. For a boy of fifteen or sixteen and upwards the boarding-school system may have its advantages. By that time a boy is old enough to understand some questions; he is old enough to have some rational ideal of conduct, and to hold his own in the pursuit of it; and he may learn in the life away from home a lot in the way of discipline, organization, self-reliance, etc. But to send a young thing, ignorant of life, and quite unformed of character, to take his chance by day and night in the public school as it at present exists, is—to say the least—a rash thing to do.]

kind are difficult; but masters are greatly hampered by the confusion in the public mind, to which we have already alluded—which so often persists in setting down any attachment between two boys, or between a boy and his teacher, to nothing but sensuality. Many masters quite understand the situation, but feel themselves helpless in the face of public opinion. Who so fit (they sometimes feel) to enlighten a young boy and guide his growing mind as one of themselves, when the bond of attachment exists between the two? Like the writer of a letter quoted in the early part of this paper they believe that "a personal affection, almost indescribable, grows up between pupil and teacher, through which thoughts are shared and an influence created that could exist in no other way." Yet when the pupil comes along of whom all this might be true, who shows by his pleading looks the sentiment which animates him, and the profound impression which he is longing, as it were, to receive from his teacher, the latter belies himself, denies his own instinct and the boy's great need, and treats him distantly and with coldness. And why? Simply because he dreads, even while he desires it, the boy's confidence. He fears the ingenuous and perfectly natural expression of the boy's affection in caress or embrace, because he knows how a bastard public opinion will interpret, or misinterpret it; and rather than run such a risk as this he seals the fountains of the heart, withholds the help which love alone can give, and deliberately nips the tender bud which is turning to him for light and warmth. [58]

The panic terror which prevails in England with regard to the expression of affection of this kind has its comic aspect. The affection exists, and is known to exist, on all sides; but we must bury our heads in the sand and pretend not to see it. And if by any chance we are compelled to recognize it, we must show our vast discernment by SUSPECTING it. And thus we fling on the dust-heap one of the noblest and most precious elements in human nature. Certainly, if the denial and suspicion

---

[58] [Note: It should be also said, in fairness, that the fear of showing undue partiality, often comes in as a paralysing influence.]

of all natural affection were beneficial, we should find this out in our schools; but seeing how complete is its failure there to clarify their tone it is sufficiently evident that the method itself is wrong.

The remarks in this paper have chiefly had reference to boys' schools; but they apply in the main to girls' schools, where much the same troubles prevail—with this difference, that in girls' schools friendships instead of being repressed are rather encouraged by public opinion; only unfortunately they are for the most part friendships of a weak and sentimental turn, and not very healthy either in themselves or in the habits they lead to. Here too, in girls' schools, the whole subject wants facing out; friendship wants setting on a more solid and less sentimental basis; and on the subject of sex, so infinitely important to women, there needs to be sensible and consistent teaching, both public and private. Possibly the co-education of boys and girls may be of use in making boys less ashamed of their feelings, and girls more healthy in the expression of them.

At any rate the more the matter is thought of, the clearer I believe will it appear that a healthy affection must in the end be the basis of education, and that the recognition of this will form the only way out of the modern school-difficulty. It is true that such a change would revolutionise our school-life; but it will have to come, all the same, and no doubt will come pari passu with other changes that are taking place in society at large.

V

THE PLACE OF THE URANIAN IN SOCIETY

Whatever differing views there may be on the many problems which the Intermediate sexes present—and however difficult of solution some of the questions involved—there is one thing which appears to me incontestable: namely that a vast number of intermediates do actually perform most valuable social work, and that they do so partly on account and by reason of their special temperament.

This fact is not generally recognised as it ought to be, for the simple reason that the Uranian himself is not recognised, and indeed (as we have already said) tends to conceal his temperament from the public. There is no doubt that if it became widely known WHO ARE the Uranians, the world would be astonished to find so many of its great or leading men among them.

I have thought it might be useful to indicate some of the lines along which valuable work is being performed, or has been performed, by people of this disposition; and in doing this I do not of course mean to disguise or conceal the fact that there are numbers of merely frivolous, or feeble or even vicious homosexuals, who practically do no useful work for society at all—JUST AS THERE ARE OF NORMAL PEOPLE. The existence of those who do no valuable work does not alter the fact of the existence of others whose work is of great importance. And I wish also to make it clearly understood that I use the word Uranians to indicate simply those whose lives and activities are inspired by a genuine friendship or love for their own sex, without venturing to specify their individual and particular habits or relations towards those whom they love (which relations in most cases we have no means of knowing). Some Intermediates of light and leading—doubtless not a few—are physically very reserved and continent; others are sensual in some degree or other. The point is that they are all men, or women, whose most powerful motive comes from the dedication to their own kind, and is bound up with it in some way. And if it seems strange and anomalous that in such cases work of considerable importance to society is being done by people whose affections and dispositions society itself would blame, this is after all no more than has happened a thousand times before in the history of the world.

As I have already hinted, the Uranian temperament (probably from the very fact of its dual nature and the swift and constant interaction between its masculine and feminine elements) is exceedingly sensitive and emotional; and there is no doubt that, going with this, a large number of the artist class, musical, literary or pictorial, belong to this description. That delicate and subtle sympathy with every wave and phase of feeling which makes the artist possible is also very characteristic of the Uranian (the male type), and makes it easy or natural for the Uranian man to become an artist. In the "confessions" and "cases" collected by Krafft-Ebing, Havelock Ellis and others, it is remarkable what a large percentage of men of this temperament belong to the artist class. In his volume on "Sexual Inversion,"[59] speaking of the cases collected by himself, Ellis says:—"An examination of my cases reveals the interesting fact that thirty- two of them, or sixty-eight per cent., possess artistic aptitude in varying degree. Galton found, from the investigation of nearly one thousand persons, that the general average showing artistic taste in England is only about thirty per cent. It must also be said that my figures are probably below the truth, as no special point was made of investigating the matter, and also that in many of my cases the artistic aptitudes are of high order. With regard to the special avocations of my cases, it must of course be said that no occupation furnishes a safeguard against inversion. There are, however, certain occupations to which inverts are specially attracted. Acting is certainly one of the chief of these. Three of my cases belong to the dramatic profession, and others have marked dramatic ability. Art, again, in its various forms, and music, exercise much attraction. In my experience, however, literature is the avocation to which inverts seem to feel chiefly

---

[59] [Note: "Studies in the Psychology of Sex," vol. ii., p. 173.]

called, and that moreover in which they may find the highest degree of success and reputation. At least half-a-dozen of my cases are successful men of letters."

Of Literature in this connection, and of the great writers of the world whose work has been partly inspired by the Uranian love, I have myself already spoken.[60] It may further be said that those of the modern artist-writers and poets who have done the greatest service in the way of interpreting and reconstructing Greek life and ideals—men like Winckelmann, Goethe, Addington Symonds, Walter Pater—have had a marked strain of this temperament in them. And this has been a service of great value, and one which the world could ill have afforded to lose.

The painters and sculptors, especially of the renaissance period in Italy, yield not a few examples of men whose work has been similarly inspired—as in the cases of Michel Angelo, Leonardo, Bazzi, Cellini, and others. As to music, this is certainly the art which in its subtlety and tenderness—and perhaps in a certain inclination to INDULGE in emotion—lies nearest to the Urning nature. There are few in fact of this nature who have not some gift in the direction of music—though, unless we cite Tschaikowsky, it does not appear that any thorough-going Uranian has attained to the highest eminence in this art.

Another direction along which the temperament very naturally finds an outlet is the important social work of Education. The capacity that a man has, in cases, of devoting himself to the welfare of boys or youths, is clearly a thing which ought not to go wasted—and which may be most precious and valuable. It is incontestable that a great number of men (and women) are drawn into the teaching profession by this sentiment—and the work they do is, in many cases, beyond estimation. Fortunate the boy who meets with such a helper in early life! I know a man—a rising and vigorous thinker and writer—who tells me that he owes almost everything mentally to such a friend of his boyhood, who took the greatest interest

[60] [Note: See ch. ii. supra, also Ioläus, an Anthology of Friendship, by E. Carpenter.]

in him, saw him almost every day for many years, and indeed cleared up for him not only things mental but things moral, giving him the affection and guidance his young heart needed. And I have myself known and watched not a few such teachers, in public schools and in private schools, and seen something of the work and of the real inspiration they have been to boys under them. Hampered as they have been by the readiness of the world to misinterpret, they still have been able to do most precious service. Of course here and there a case occurs in which privilege is abused; but even then the judgment of the world is often unreasonably severe. A poor boy once told me with tears in his eyes of the work a man had done for him. This man had saved the boy from drunken parents, taken him from the slums, and by means of a club helped him out into the world. Many other boys he had rescued, it appeared, in the same way—scores and scores of them. But on some occasion or other he got into trouble, and was accused of improper familiarities. No excuse, or record of a useful life, was of the least avail. Every trumpery slander was believed, every mean motive imputed, and he had to throw up his position and settle elsewhere, his life-work shattered, never to be resumed.

The capacity for sincere affection which causes an elder man to care so deeply for the welfare of a youth or boy, is met and responded to by a similar capacity in the young thing of devotion to an elder man. This fact is not always recognised; but I have known cases of boys and even young men who would feel the most romantic attachments to quite mature men, sometimes as much as forty or fifty years of age, and only for them—passing by their own contemporaries of either sex, and caring only to win a return affection from these others. This may seem strange, but it is true. And the fact not only makes one understand what riddles there are slumbering in the breasts of our children, but how greatly important it is that we should try to read them—since here, in such cases as these, the finding of an answering heart in an elder man would probably be the younger one's salvation.

How much of the enormous amount of philanthropic work done in the present day—by women among needy or destitute girls of all sorts, or by men among like classes of boys—is inspired by the same feeling, it would be hard to say; but it must be a very considerable proportion. I think myself that the best philanthropic work—just because it is the most personal, the most loving, and the least merely formal and self-righteous—has a strong fibre of the Uranian heart running through it; and if it should be said that work of this very personal kind is more liable to dangers and difficulties on that account, it is only what is true of the best in almost all departments.

Eros is a great leveller. Perhaps the true Democracy rests, more firmly than anywhere else, on a sentiment which easily passes the bounds of class and caste, and unites in the closest affection the most estranged ranks of society. It is noticeable how often Uranians of good position and breeding are drawn to rougher types, as of manual workers, and frequently very permanent alliances grow up in this way, which although not publicly acknowledged have a decided influence on social institutions, customs and political tendencies—and which would have a good deal more influence could they be given a little more scope and recognition. There are cases that I have known (although the ordinary commercial world might hardly believe it) of employers who have managed to attach their workmen, or many of them, very personally to themselves, and whose object in running their businesses was at least as much to provide their employees with a living as themselves; while the latter, feeling this, have responded with their best output. It is possible that something like the guilds and fraternities of the middle ages might thus be reconstructed, but on a more intimate and personal basis than in those days; and indeed there are not wanting signs that such a reconstruction is actually taking place.

The "Letters of Love and Labour" written by Samuel M. Jones of Toledo, Ohio, to his workmen in the engineering firm of which he was master, are very interesting in this connection. They breathe a spirit of extraordinary personal affection towards, and confidence in, the employees, which was heartily responded to by the latter; and the whole business was carried on, with considerable success, on the principle of a close and friendly co- operation all round. [61]

These things indeed suggest to one that it is possible that the Uranian spirit may lead to something like a general enthusiasm of Humanity, and that the Uranian people may be destined to form the advance guard of that great movement which will one day transform the common life by substituting the bond of personal affection and compassion for the monetary, legal and other external ties which now control and confine society. Such a part of course we cannot expect the Uranians to play unless the capacity for their kind of attachment also exists—though in a germinal and undeveloped state— in the breast of mankind at large. And modern thought and investigation are clearly tending that way—to confirm that it does so exist.

Dr. E. Bertz in his late study of Whitman as a person of strongly homogenic temperament [62] brings forward the objection that Whitman's gospel of Comradeship as a means of social regeneration is founded on a false basis—because (so Dr. Bertz says) the gospel derives from an abnormality in himself, and therefore cannot possibly have a universal application or create a general enthusiasm. But this is rather a case of assuming the point which has to be proved. Whitman constantly maintains that his own disposition at any rate is normal, and that he represents the average man. And it MAY be true, even as far as his Uranian temperament is concerned, that while this was specially developed in him the germs of it ARE almost, if not quite, universal. If so, then the Comradeship on which Whitman founds a large portion of his message may in course of time become a general enthusiasm, and the nobler Uranians of to-day may be destined, as suggested, to be its pioneers and advance guard. As one of them himself has sung:—

---

[61] [Note: Mr. Jones became Mayor of Toledo; but died at the early age of 53. See also "Workshop Reconstruction," by C. R. Ashbee, Appendix, intra, p. 146.]

[62] [Note: "Whitman: ein Charakterbild," by Edward Bertz (Leipzig, Max Spohr).]

These things shall be! A loftier race,
  Than e'er the world hath known, shall rise
With flame of freedom in their souls,
  And light of science in their eyes.
Nation with nation, land with land,
  In-armed shall live as comrades free;
In every heart and brain shall throb
  The pulse of one fraternity.[63]

To proceed. The Uranian, though generally high-strung and sensitive, is by no means always dreamy. He is sometimes extraordinarily and unexpectedly practical; and such a man may, and often does, command a positive enthusiasm among his subordinates in a business organisation. The same is true of military organisation. As a rule the Uranian temperament (in the male) is not militant. War with its horrors and savagery is somewhat alien to the type. But here again there are exceptions; and in all times there have been great generals (like Alexander, Cæsar, Charles XII. of Sweden, or Frederick II. of Prussia—not to speak of more modern examples) with a powerful strain in them of the homogenic nature, and a wonderful capacity for organisation and command, which combined with their personal interest in, or attachment to, their troops, and the answering enthusiasm so elicited, have made their armies well-nigh invincible.

The existence of this great practical ability in some Uranians cannot be denied; and it points to the important work they may some day have to do in social reconstruction. At the same time I think it is noticeable that POLITICS (at any rate in the modern sense of the word, as concerned mainly with party questions and party government) is not as a rule congenial to them. The personal and affectional element is perhaps too remote or absent. Mere "views" and "questions" and party strife are alien to the Uranian man, as they are on the whole to the ordinary woman.

---

[63] [Note: John Addington Symonds.]

If politics, however, are not particularly congenial, it is yet remarkable how many royal personages have been decidedly homogenic in temperament. Taking the Kings of England from the Norman Conquest to the present day, we may count about thirty. And three of these, namely, William Rufus, Edward II., and James I. were homosexual in a marked degree—might fairly be classed as Urnings— while some others, like William III., had a strong admixture of the same temperament. Three out of thirty yields a high ratio—ten per cent—and considering that sovereigns do not generally choose themselves, but come into their position by accident of birth, the ratio is certainly remarkable. Does it suggest that the general percentage in the world at large is equally high, but that it remains unnoticed, except in the fierce light that beats upon thrones? or is there some other explanation with regard to the special liability of royalty to inversion? Hereditary degeneracy has sometimes been suggested. But it is difficult to explain the matter even on this theory; for though the epithet "degenerate" might possibly apply to James I., it would certainly not be applicable to William Rufus and William III., who, in their different ways, were both men of great courage and personal force— while Edward II. was by no means wanting in ability.

But while the Uranian temperament has, in cases, specially fitted its possessors to become distinguished in art or education or war or administration, and enabled them to do valuable work in these fields; it remains perhaps true that above all it has fitted them, and fits them, for distinction and service in affairs of the heart.

It is hard to imagine human beings more skilled in these matters than are the Intermediates. For indeed no one else can possibly respond to and understand, as they do, all the fluctuations and interactions of the masculine and feminine in human life. The pretensive coyness and passivity of women, the rude invasiveness of men; lust, brutality, secret tears, the bleeding heart; renunciation, motherhood, finesse, romance, angelic devotion—all these things lie slumbering in the Uranian soul, ready on occasion for expression; and if they are not always expressed are always there for purposes of divination or interpretation. There are few situations, in fact, in courtship or marriage which the Uranian does not instinctively understand; and it is strange to see how even an unlettered person of this type will often read Love's manuscript easily in cases where the normal man or woman is groping over it like a child in the dark. [Not of course that this means to imply any superiority of CHARACTER in the former; but merely that with his double outlook he necessarily discerns things which the other misses.]

That the Uranians do stand out as helpers and guides, not only in matters of Education, but in affairs of love and marriage, is tolerably patent to all who know them. It is a common experience for them to be consulted now by the man, now by the woman, whose matrimonial conditions are uncongenial or disastrous—not generally because the consultants in the least perceive the Uranian nature, but because they instinctively feel that here is a strong sympathy with and understanding of their side of the question. In this way it is often the fate of the Uranian, himself unrecognised, to bring about happier times and a better comprehension of each other among those with whom he may have to deal. Also he often becomes the confidant of young things of either sex, who are caught in the tangles of love or passion, and know not where to turn for assistance.

I say that I think perhaps of all the services the Uranian may render to society it will be found some day that in this direction of solving the problems of affection and of the heart he will do the greatest service. If the day is coming as we have suggested— when Love is at last to take its rightful place as the binding and directing force of society (instead of the Cash-nexus), and society is to be transmuted in consequence to a higher form, then undoubtedly the superior types of Uranians—prepared for this service by long experience and devotion, as well as by much suffering—will have an important part to play in the transformation. For that the Urnings in their own lives put Love before everything else—postponing to it the other motives like money-making, business success, fame, which occupy so much space in most people's careers—is a fact which is patent to everyone who knows them. This may be saying little or nothing in favour of those of this class whose conception of love is only of a poor and frivolous sort; but in the case of those others who see the god in his true light, the fact that they serve him in singleness of heart and so unremittingly raises them at once into the position of the natural leaders of mankind.

From this fact—i.e., that these folk think so much of affairs of the heart—and from the fact that their alliances and friendships are formed and carried on beneath the surface of society, as it were, and therefore to some extent beyond the inquisitions and supervisions of Mrs. Grundy, some interesting conclusions flow.

For one thing, the question is constantly arising as to how Society would shape itself if FREE: what form, in matters of Love and Marriage, it would take, if the present restrictions and sanctions were removed or greatly altered. At present in these matters, the Law, the Church, and a strong pressure of public opinion interfere, compelling the observance of certain forms; and it becomes difficult to say how much of the existing order is due to the spontaneous instinct and common sense of human nature, and how much to mere outside compulsion and interference: how far, for instance, Monogamy is natural or artificial; to what degree marriages would be permanent if the Law did not make them so; what is the rational view of Divorce; whether jealousy is a necessary accompaniment of Love; and so forth. These are questions which are being constantly discussed, without finality; or not infrequently with quite pessimistic conclusions.

Now in the Urning societies a certain freedom (though not complete, of course) exists. Underneath the surface of general Society, and consequently unaffected to any great degree by its laws and customs, alliances are formed and maintained, or modified or broken, more in accord with inner need than with outer pressure. Thus it happens that in these societies there are such opportunities to note and observe human grouping under conditions of freedom, as do not occur in the ordinary world. And the results are both interesting and encouraging. As a rule I think it may be said that the alliances are remarkably permanent. Instead of the wild "general post" which so many good people seem to expect in the event of law being relaxed, one finds (except of course in a few individual cases) that common sense and fidelity and a strong tendency to permanence prevail. In the ordinary world so far has doubt gone that many to-day disbelieve in a life-long free marriage. Yet among the Uranians such a thing is, one may almost say, common and well known; and there are certainly few among them who do not believe in its possibility.

Great have been the debates, in all times and places, concerning Jealousy; and as to how far jealousy is natural and instinctive and universal, and how far it is the product of social opinion and the property sense, and so on. In ordinary marriage what may be called social and proprietary jealousy is undoubtedly a very great factor. But this kind of jealousy hardly appears or operates in the Urning societies. Thus we have an opportunity in these latter of observing conditions where only the natural and instinctive jealousy exists. This of course is present among the Urnings— sometimes rampant and violent, sometimes quiescent and vanishing almost to nil. It seems to depend almost entirely upon the individual; and we certainly learn that jealousy, though frequent and widespread, is not an absolutely necessary accompaniment of love. There are cases of Uranians (whether men or women) who, though permanently allied, do not object to lesser friendships on either side—and there are cases of very decided objection. And we may conclude that something the same would be true (is true) of the ordinary Marriage, the property considerations and the property jealousy being once removed. The tendency anyhow to establish a dual relation more or less fixed, is seen to be very strong among the Intermediates, and may be concluded to be equally strong among the more normal folk.

Again with regard to Prostitution. That there are a few natural- born prostitutes is seen in the Urning-societies; but prostitution in that world does not take the important place which it does in the normal world, partly because the law-bound compulsory marriage does not exist there, and partly because prostitution naturally has little chance and cannot compete in a world where alliances are free and there is an open field for friendship. Hence we may see that freedom of alliance and of marriage in the ordinary world will probably lead to the great diminution or even disappearance of Prostitution.

In these and other ways the experience of the Uranian world forming itself freely and not subject to outside laws and institutions comes as a guide—and really a hopeful guide—towards the future. I would say however that in making these remarks about certain conclusions which we are able to gather from some spontaneous and comparatively unrestricted associations, I do not at all mean to argue AGAINST institutions and forms. I think that the Uranian love undoubtedly suffers from want of a recognition and a standard. And though it may at present be better off than if subject to a foolish and meddlesome regulation; yet in the future it will have its more or less fixed standards and ideals, like the normal love. If one considers for a moment how the ordinary relations of the sexes would suffer were there no generally acknowledged codes of honour and conduct with regard to them, one then indeed sees that reasonable forms and institutions are a help, and one may almost wonder that the Urning circles are so well-conducted on the whole as they are.

I have said that the Urning men in their own lives put love before money-making, business success, fame, and other motives which rule the normal man. I am sure that it is also true of them as a whole that they put love before lust. I do not feel SURE that this can be said of the normal man, at any rate in the present stage of evolution. It is doubtful whether on the whole the merely physical attraction is not the stronger motive with the latter type. Unwilling as the world at large is to credit what I am about to say, and great as are the current misunderstandings on the subject, I believe it is true that the Uranian men are superior to the normal men in this respect—in respect of their love-feeling—which is gentler, more sympathetic, more considerate, more a matter of the heart and less one of mere physical satisfaction than that of ordinary men.[64] All this flows naturally from the presence of the feminine element in them, and its blending with the rest of their nature. It should be expected a priori, and it can be noticed at once by those who have any acquaintance with the Urning world. Much of the current misunderstanding with

---

[64] [Note: See Appendix, pp. 172-174.]

regard to the character and habits of the Urning arises from his confusion with the ordinary roué who, though of normal temperament, contracts homosexual habits out of curiosity and so forth—but this is a point which I have touched on before, and which ought now to be sufficiently clear. If it be once allowed that the love-nature of the Uranian is of a sincere and essentially humane and kindly type then the importance of the Uranian's place in Society, and of the social work he may be able to do, must certainly also be acknowledged.

APPENDIX

"In this country [Britain] we have too long, from a sense of mock modesty, neglected the science relating to sex. In Germany this is not so. There we find workers who have elaborated for themselves a new science, and who have given to the world knowledge which is of the very utmost importance. We now know that there are females with strong male characteristics and vice-versa. Anatomically and mentally we find all shades existing from the pure genus man to the pure genus woman. Thus there has been constituted what is well named by an illustrious exponent of the science 'The Third Sex'."— Dr. JAMES BURNET, The Medical Times and Hospital Gazette, vol. xxxiv., No. 1497, 10th November, 1906. London.

"Every citizen of age to fulfil his duties as a citizen, whether he be a father or husband, teacher or pupil, master or servant, official or subordinate, has the right, and owes it as a duty, to know the facts of sexual inversion, to combat and to prevent debauchery, crime and vice, to learn and to teach others the place of inversion in Society, and its morals, the duties of the invert towards himself, and towards other inverts, towards the normal man, and towards women and children. And the duties of the normal man towards the invert are no less—no less difficult, no less indispensable."—M. A. RAFFALOVICH, "Uranisme et Unisexualité." Paris, 1896.

"That sex inversion is not a chance phenomenon . . . appears from the fact that it has been observed at all times and in all places, and among peoples quite separate from each other."—A. MOLL, "Die Konträre Sexualempfindung," 2nd Edition, p. 15. Berlin, 1893.

"Concerning the wide prevalence of sexual inversion, and of homosexual phenomena generally, there can be no manner of doubt. In Berlin, Moll states that he has himself seen between six hundred and seven hundred homosexual persons, and heard of some two hundred and fifty to three hundred others. I have much evidence as to its frequency both in England and the United States. In England, concerning which I can naturally speak with most assurance, its manifestations are well-marked for those whose eyes have been opened. . . . Among the professional and most cultured element of the middle class in England there must be a distinct percentage of inverts, which may sometimes be as much as five per cent., though such estimates must always be hazardous. Among women of the same class the percentage seems to be at least double—though here the phenomena are less definite and deep-seated."—HAVELOCK ELLIS, "Psychology of Sex," vol. Sexual Inversion, pp. 29, 30. Philadelphia, 1901.

———

"According to the information of De Joux in 'The Disinherited of Love,' the number of Urnings in all Europe is about five millions; about 4.5 per cent. of all males in Europe are Urnings, while only 0.1 per cent. of females are Urningins. A malady therefore—if malady it should be called—which is so widespread certainly demands our deepest interest; and it is strange that it is only since the '70's that this subject has been discussed in scientific literature.

"It is owing to this ignorance that the public mind has been dominated, and still is dominated, by the prejudice, that psychical hermaphroditism and sex-inversion are nothing but crimes, wilful crimes, whereas they proceed necessarily out of the inborn nature of such individuals."—NORBERT GRABOWSKY, "Die verkehrte Geschlechtsempfindung," p. 16. Leipzig, 1894.

———

Dr. HIRSCHFELD, in his "Statistischen Untersuchunge über den Prozentensatz der Homosexuellen," gives the result of various statistical investigations on this subject; and their remarkable agreement enables him to speak with some confidence. He says (p. 41), "Now we KNOW that we must reckon the numbers of those who vary from the normal, not by fractions of thousands but by fractions of hundreds. The fact that, as a result of these various enquiries and commissions about the same figure has emerged (for the proportion of exclusively homosexual persons), namely, a figure in the neighbourhood of 1 1/2 per cent.—this extraordinary agreement cannot possibly be a chance, but must rest on a law—a law of nature—namely, that only 90 to 95 per cent. of mankind are normally sexual by birth; that about 1 1/2 to 2 per cent. are born pure homosexuals (say about 1,000,000 in Germany); and that between the two classes there remain some 4 per cent. who are bisexual by nature."

And again (p. 60), "But what do these figures show? They show that of 100,000 inhabitants on the average only 94,600 are sexually normal, while 5,400 vary from the normal. Of these latter 1,500 are exclusively homosexual, and 3,900 bisexual. While of these last again 700 are PREDOMINANTLY homosexual; so that of 100,000 Germans, 2,200 (or 2.2 per cent.) are either exclusively or predominantly homosexual— making 1,200,000 for the whole German Fatherland."

———

"Sexual inversion has usually been regarded as psycho-pathological, as a symptom of degeneration; and those who exhibit it have been considered as physically unfit. This view, however, is falling into disrepute, especially as Krafft-Ebing, its principal champion, abandoned it in the later editions of his work. None the less, it is not generally recognised that sexual inverts may be otherwise perfectly healthy, and with regard to other social matters quite normal. When they have been asked if they would have wished matters to be different with them in this respect, they almost invariably answer in the negative."— O. WEININGER, "Sex and Character," ch. iv. Heinemann, London, 1906.

———

"It is a common belief that a male who experiences love for his own sex must be despicable, degraded, depraved, vicious, and incapable of humane or generous sentiments. If Greek history did not contradict this supposition, a little patient enquiry into contemporary manners would suffice to remove it."—J. ADDINGTON SYMONDS, "A Problem in Modern Ethics," p. 10.

———

"Mantegazza rightly insists that Urnings are found by no means only among the dregs of the people, but that they are rather to be noted in circles which in respect of culture, wealth, and social position rank among the first. Thus, among the aristocracy without doubt a great number of Urnings are to be found."—A. MOLL, op. cit., p. 76.

———

"In no rank are there so many Urnings as among servants. One may say that every third male domestic is an Urning."—DE JOUX, "Die Enterbten des Liebesglückes," p. 193. Leipzig, 1893.

———

"It is therefore certain, as we have seen, that many Urnings come from nervous or pathologically disposed families. . . . All the same, I must say that there is no proof to hand in ALL cases of sex- inversion among men, that the individuals concerned are thus hereditarily weighted. And besides, there is the consideration that the extension, according to some authors, of hereditary trouble is at present so great that one may prove a tendency to nervous or mental maladies in almost everybody."—A. MOLL, op. cit., p. 221.

———

"The truth is that we can no more explain the inverted sex-feeling than we can the normal impulse; all attempts at explanation of these things, and of Love, are defective."—Ibid, p. 253.

———

"Among the PENCHANTS of Urnings one finds not infrequently a great partiality for Art and Music—and indeed, for active interest in the same as well as passive enjoyment. . . . the Actor's talent is especially noticeable among some . . . But it must not be thought that Urnings are only capable of a special activity of the imagination. On the contrary, there are undoubted cases in which they contribute something in the scientific direction . . . Also in Poetry do Urnings occasionally show exceptional talent; especially in love-verses addressed to men."—Ibid, p. 80.

———

"An examination of my cases [of Inverts] reveals the interesting fact that 68 per cent. possess artistic aptitude in varying degree. Galton found, from the investigation of nearly 1,000 persons, that the average showing artistic tastes in England is only about 30 per cent."—HAVELOCK ELLIS, "Sexual Inversion," p. 173.

_____

"In Antiquity, especially among the Greeks, there seem to have been numbers of men who in their emotional natures were hermaphrodites. I think that the study of psychical hermaphrodisy is most important, and will throw yet greater light on the psychology of Love itself. Observation so far already shows that the same individual at differing times can experience quite different sexual feelings."—A. MOLL, op. cit., p. 200.

_____

"The Urning is capable, through the force of his love, of making the greatest sacrifices for his beloved, and on that account the love of the Urning has been often compared with Woman's love. Just as the Woman's love is stronger and more devoted than that of the normal man, just as it exceeds that of the Man in inwardness, so, according to Ulrichs should the Urning's love in this respect stand higher than that of the woman-loving Man."—Ibid, p. 118.

_____

"Womanish men often know how to treat women better than manly men do. Manly men, except in most rare cases, learn how to deal with women only after long experience, and even then most imperfectly."— O. WEININGER, "Sex and Character," ch. v.

_____

"Is it really the case that all women and men are marked off sharply from each other, the women on the one hand alike in all points, the men on the other? . . . There are transitional forms between the metals and non-metals, between chemical combinations and simple mixtures, between animals and plants, between phanerogams and cryptogams, and between mammals and birds . . . The improbability may henceforth be taken for granted of finding in Nature a sharp cleavage between all that is masculine on the one side and all that is feminine on the other; or that any living being is so simple in this respect that it can be put wholly on one side, or wholly on the other, of the line."—WEININGER, Ibid, introduction, p. 2.

"Upon this, Chéron made a rather strange observation. 'We have,' she said, 'with regard to sexual distinctions, notions that were not dreamed of by the primitive simplicity of the people of the age now gone by. From the fact that there are two sexes, and only two, they for a long time drew false inferences. They concluded that a woman is simply a woman, and a man simply a man. In reality this is not so; there are women who are very much women, and women who are very little so. Such differences, concealed in former times by costume and mode of life, and masked by prejudice, stand out clearly in our society. And not only so, but they become more accentuated and apparent in each generation.'"—ANATOLE FRANCE, "Sur la Pierre Blanche," p. 301.

"In EVERY human being there are present both male and female elements, only in normal persons (according to their sex) the one set of elements is more greatly developed than the other. The chief difference in the case of homosexual persons is that in them the male and female elements are more equalized; so that when, in addition, the general development is of a high grade, we find among this class the most perfect types of humanity."—Dr. ARDUIN, "Die Frauenfrage," in Jahrbuch der Sexuellen Zwischenstufen, vol. ii., p. 217. Leipzig, 1900.

"The notion that human beings were originally hermaphroditic is both ancient and widespread. We find it in the book of Genesis, unless indeed there be a confusion here between two separate theories of creation. God is said to have first made man in His image, male and female in one body, and to have bidden them multiply. Later on He created the woman out of part of this primitive man." (See also the myth related by Aristophanes in Plato's Symposium.)—HAVELOCK ELLIS, "Sexual Inversion," p. 229.

"When the sexual instinct first appears in early youth, it seems to be much less specialised than normally it becomes later. Not only is it, at the outset, less definitely directed to a specific sexual end, but even the sex of its object is sometimes uncertain." Ibid, p. 44.

———

"In me the homosexual nature is singularly complete, and is undoubtedly congenital. The most intense delight of my childhood (even when a tiny boy in my nurse's charge) was to watch acrobats and riders at the circus. This was not so much for the skilful feats as on account of the beauty of their persons. Even then I cared chiefly for the more lithe and graceful fellows. People told me that circus actors were wicked and would steal little boys, and so I came to look on my favourites as half-devil and half-angel. When I was older and could go about alone, I would often hang around the tents of travelling shows in hope of catching a glimpse of the actors. I longed to see them naked, without their tights, and used to lie awake at night, thinking of them and longing to be embraced and loved by them."—Ibid, "case" ix., p. 62.

———

"I was fifteen years and ten-and-a-half months old when the first erotic dream announced the arrival of puberty. I had had no previous experience of sex-satisfaction, either in the Urning direction or in any other. This occurrence therefore came about quite normally. From a much earlier time, however, I had been subject partly to tender yearnings and partly to sensual longing without definite form and purpose—the two emotions being always separate from each other and never experienced for one and the same young man. These aimless sensual longings plagued me often in hours of solitude; and I could not overcome them. They showed themselves first, during my fifteenth year, when I was at school at Detmold, in the following two ways:—First, they were awakened by a drawing in Normand's 'Saülenordnungen,' of the figure of a Greek god or hero, standing there in naked beauty. This image, a hundred times put away, came again a hundred times before my mind. (I need not say it did not CAUSE the Urning temperament in me; it merely awoke what was slumbering there already—a thing that any other circumstance might have done.) Secondly, when studying in my little room, or when I lay upon my bed before going to sleep, the thought used suddenly and irresistibly to rise up in my mind—'If only a soldier would clamber through the window and come into my room!' Then my imagination painted me a splendid soldier- figure of twenty to twenty-two years old; and I was, as it were, all on fire. And yet my thoughts were quite vague, and undirected to any definite satisfaction; nor had I ever spoken a word with a real soldier."—K. H. ULRICHS, "Memnon," § 77. Leipzig, 1898. See also "A Problem in Modern Ethics," p. 73.

———

"The friendships of this kind which I formed at School were two in number—I shall never forget the absorbing depth and intensity of them. I never talked about them to anyone else, they were much too sacred and serious for that, nor—strange as it may seem—did I ever speak of them to the boys themselves, or indeed, show any signs of affection towards them. If they had been told that I was devoted to their welfare, and willing to sacrifice myself and all I had to it (which was indeed the fact) they would have been simply astonished; more especially as they were both young boys not yet arrived at puberty.

"I am at present somewhat bitterly conscious that in these cases one of the strongest influences for good that ever came into my life was nine-tenths wasted. How much better it all might have been under more favourable surroundings it is impossible to imagine. Still, it was not without its good influence on me, though (owing to their complete ignorance of my feelings) it could have had none whatever on the boys. I was conscious of a bracing and inspiring effect on my whole nature, a confirmed health of body, and most of all, of a greatly increased capacity for work. And doubtless all this might have been intensified a thousand fold if I had been ever so little guided and encouraged by public opinion sanctioning these friendships.

"The Public School boy has after all strong feelings of honour and fairness: and I am sure much might be done by cultivating the Public Opinion of the school: making devoted and disinterested friendships highly thought of and praised, and condemning as base and mean the least attempt to befoul a young boy's purity through a gross and selfish desire for personal gratification. School public opinion would, I am sure, tend quite readily to flow in such channels. But this would demand an openness of treatment of the whole question such as does not at present exist. That the greatest force the schoolmaster has at his command should be so ignored (and so needlessly) is more than absurd: it is monstrous. And it concerns him as a teacher quite as much as the boys themselves in their relations with each other. I believe that gaining a boy's affection is the necessary preliminary to really TEACHING him anything. Otherwise you do not really teach him at all."— Private letter.

___

"I could tell you a good deal of another equally strong friendship I formed (myself twenty-five, boy fourteen) which was one of the happiest events of my life. It was acknowledged on both sides, but perfectly restrained and pure: and we saw a great deal of each other during most of the school holidays for about a year. I could have done anything with that boy, my influence over him was for the time being I should say unlimited: and undoubtedly IMMENSE good accrued to us both."—Ibid.

___

"In my own school-life—as a day scholar—I had two such friendships, though of course in a day school there was not the same possibility of their development. One was with an elder boy some five years my senior, and the other with a master some twelve years older than myself. I was a shy, timid youngster, and not having a robust physique did not enter much into the ordinary athletics of the school. My elder friend was a very delicate, gentle, refined boy with a purity and loftiness of mind in striking contrast to the filthy moral atmosphere of the school at that time, but he was never censorious or self-righteous. I feel that this friendship was the most powerful influence in my early life in keeping a high ideal of conduct before me—much more powerful than the influence of home, which I do not think I was at all conscious of.

"After he left school, for Cambridge, we used to write regularly to one another—long letters, hardly ever less than three sheets in length. I remember I used to think him the most handsome man I knew, but looking now at his photo taken about that time and comparing it with others, I see that his features were inferior to many others of my school-fellows. At the end of his second year he died of consumption. It was during the Long Vacation, and I was abroad at the time. I remember I used to sit up late into the night writing very long letters to him about all I had seen, to interest him during his illness. I did not know how ill he really was, but I had a terrible fear that I should not see him again. When I got back and found he had just died the shock was awful. For weeks I felt as if I had not a friend in the whole world. I have never felt any loss so keenly either before or since. . . .

"The other friendship with my mathematical master, though not so intimate, was still of a very affectionate character. I feel I owe a great deal to it—he laid the foundation of my ideal of a teacher's duty to his pupils."—Private letter.

———

"It is not new in itself; this, the feeling that drew Jesus to John, or Shakespeare to the youth of the sonnets, or that inspired the friendships of Greece, has been with us before, and in the new citizenship we shall need it again. The Whitmanic love of comrades is its modern expression; Democracy—as socially, not politically conceived—its basis. The thought as to how much of the solidarity of labour and the modern Trade-Union movement may be due to an unconscious faith in this principle of comradeship, is no idle one. The freer, more direct, and more genuine relationship between men, which is implied by it, must be the ultimate basis of the reconstructed Workshop."—C. R. ASHBEE, "Workshop Reconstruction and Citizenship," p. 160.

———

A case of passionate attachment between two Indian boys was told to the author of the present book by a master at a school in India. The boys—who were about sixteen years of age—were both at the same school, and were devoted friends; but the day came when they had to part. One was taken away by his parents to go to a distant part of the country. The other was inconsolable at the prospect. When the day arrived, and his companion was removed, he soon after went quietly to a well in the school precincts, jumped in, and was drowned. The news, sent on by wire, reached the departing friend while still on his journey. He said little, but at one of the stations left the train and disappeared. The train went on, but at a little distance out, the boy ran out of the bushes by the line, threw himself on the rails, and was killed.

———

The following is taken from one of the "cases" recorded by Havelock Ellis in his "Sexual Inversion": "The earliest sex-impression that I am conscious of is at the age of nine or ten falling in love with a handsome boy who must have been about two years my senior. I do not recollect ever having spoken to him, but my desire, as far as I can recall, was that he should seize hold of and handle me. I have a distinct impression yet of how pleasurable even physical pain or cruelty would have been at his hands."—HAVELOCK ELLIS, op. cit., "case" xiii., p. 71.

———

"When I was about sixteen-and-a-half years old, there came into the house a boy about two years younger than myself, who became the absorbing thought of my school-days. I do not remember a moment, from the time I first saw him to the time I left school, that I was not in love with him, and the affection was reciprocated, if somewhat reservedly. He was always a little ahead of me in books and scholarship, but as our affection ripened we spent most of our spare time together, and he received my advances much as a girl who is being wooed, a little mockingly perhaps, but with real pleasure. He allowed me to fondle and caress him, but our intimacy never went further than a kiss, and about that even was the slur of shame; there was always a barrier between us, and we never so much as whispered to one another concerning those things of which all the school obscenely talked."—Same case, p. 73.

———

"At the age of twenty-one I began gradually to remark that I was somehow not like my comrades, that I had no pleasure in male occupations, that smoking, drinking, and card-playing gave me little satisfaction, and that I had a real death-horror of a brothel. And as a matter of fact, I had never been in one, as on every occasion under some pretext or other I have succeeded in stealing off. I now began to think about myself; I felt myself frightfully desolate, miserable and unfortunate, and longed for a friend of the same nature as myself—yet without dreaming that there could be other such men. At the age of twenty-two I came to know a young man who at last cleared up my mind about sexual inversion and those affected with it, since he—an Urning, like myself—had fallen in love with me. The scales fell from my eyes, and I bless the day which brought light to me. . . . Towards woman in her sexual relation I feel a real horror, which the exercise of all my strongest powers of imagination would not avail to overcome; and indeed, I have never attempted to overcome it, since I am quite persuaded of the fruitlessness of such an attempt, which to me appears sinful and unnatural."—KRAFFT-EBING, "Psychopathia Sexualis," 7th edition, "case" No. 122, p. 291. Stuttgart, 1892.

———

"I can no longer exist without men's love; without such I must ever remain at strife with myself. . . . If marriage between men existed I believe I should not be afraid of a lifelong union—a thing which with a woman seems to be something impossible. . . . Since, however, this kind of love is reckoned criminal, by its satisfaction I can be at harmony with myself but never with the world, and necessarily in consequence must ever be somewhat out of tune; and all the more so because my character is open, and I hate lies of all kinds. This torment, to have always to conceal everything, has forced me to confess my anomaly to a few friends, of whose understanding and reticence I am sure. Although oftentimes my condition seems to me sad enough, by reason of the difficulty of satisfaction and the general contempt of manly love, yet I am often just a little proud on account of having these anomalous feelings. Naturally, I shall never marry—but this seems to me by no means a misfortune, although I am fond of family life, and up to now have passed my time only among my own relations. I live in the hope that later I shall have a permanent loved one; such indeed I must have, else would the future seem gray and drear, and every object which folk usually pursue—honour, high position, etc.—only vain and unattractive.

"Should this hope not be fulfilled, I know that I should be unable, permanently and with pleasure, to give myself to my calling, and that I should be capable of setting aside everything in order to gain the love of a man. I feel no longer any moral scruples on account of my anomalous leaning, and generally have never been troubled because I felt myself drawn to youths. . . . Up to now it has only seemed to me bad and immoral to do that which is injurious to another, or which I would not wish done to myself, and in this respect I can say that I try as much as possible not to infringe on the rights of others, and am capable of being violently roused by any injustice done to others."—Ibid, p. 249, "case" No. 110 (official in a factory, age 31).

———

"My thoughts are by no means exclusively of the body or morbidly sensual. How often at the sight of a handsome youth does a deeply enthusiastic mood come upon me, and I offer a prayer, so to speak, in the glorious words of Heine—'Du bist wie eine Blume, so hold, so schön, so rein'. . . . Never has a young man yet guessed my love for him, I have never corrupted or damaged the morals of one, but for many have I here and there smoothed their pathway; and then I stick at no trouble and make sacrifices such as I can only make for them.

"When thus I have a chance to have a loved friend near me, to teach, to support and help, when my unconfest love finds a loving response (though naturally not sexual), then all the unclean images fade more and more from my mind. Then does my love become almost platonic, and lifts itself up—only to sink again in the mire, when it is deprived of its proper activity.

"For the rest, I am—and I can say it without boasting—not one of the worst of men. Mentally more sensitive than most average folk, I take interest in everything that moves mankind. I am kindly-disposed, tender, and easily moved to pity, can do no injury to any animal, certainly not to a human being, but on the contrary am active in a human-friendly way, where and however I can.

"Though then before my own conscience I cannot reproach myself, and though I must certainly reject the judgment of the world about us, yet I suffer greatly. In very truth I have injured no one; and I hold my love in its nobler activity for just as holy as that of normally disposed men, but under the unhappy fate that allows us neither sufferance nor recognition, I suffer often more than my life can bear."—Ibid, p. 268, "case" No. 114.

———

"To depict all the misery, all the unfortunate situations, the constant dread of being found out in one's peculiarity and of becoming impossible in society—to give an idea of all this is truly more than pen or words can compass. The very thought, so soon as it arises, of losing one's social existence and of being rejected by everybody is more torment than can be imagined. In such a case, everything, everything would be forgotten that one had ever done in the way of good; in the consciousness of his lofty morality every normally disposed man would puff himself up, however frivolously he might really have acted in the matter of his love. I know many such normal folk whose unworthy conception of their love is indeed hard for me to understand."—Ibid, p. 269.

———

"The torturing images of betrayed love prevent my sleeping, so that I am forced, now and again, to have recourse to chloral. My dreams are only a continuation of actual life, and just as painful. How all this will end I really know not; but I suppose these root- emotions must take their own course . . . The only reasonable end of the struggle is Death."—A. MOLL, "Conträre Sexualempfindung," 2nd edition, p. 123 (quotation from a letter).

———

"Weary and worn, I have passed through every tempest of anguish and despair. Years of the most racking mental agony have gone over my head without killing me. Through the long night watches I have heard the unceasing hours toll. Sleep has never been thought of by me, but I have lain on my bed trying to read some book, or have knelt by my bedside and endeavoured to raise my heart and spirit in prayer for succour or forgiveness. At last, unable to hold out any longer, with mouth tight-closed and knitted brow the Charmer has deadened my senses for one or two brief hours; but only that I may wake to a stronger and clearer perception of my hopeless condition.

"How the days have got on I know not. How I can have lived so long through such misery I know not. But torture like this is cruelly slow, whilst it is sure. It is the nature of youth to be long- enduring where Love is put to the test and a kind of occasional flicker—a kind of mocking semblance of hope, as like to hope as the rushing meteor is to the enduring sun— helps to support the load of misery, and so to prolong it. I am hundreds of years old in this my wretchedness of every moment. I cannot battle against Love and crush it out—never! God has implanted the necessity of the sentiment in my heart; it is scarce possible not to ask oneself why has He implanted so divine an element in my nature, which is doomed to die unsatisfied, which is destined in the end to be my very death?"—From a manuscript left to the Author by an Urning.

———

H. ELLIS, in Appendix D. of his book on "Sexual Inversion," speaks at some length on the School-friendships of girls: what they call "Flames" and "Raves"; of love at first sight; romance; courtship; meetings despite all obstacles; long letters; jealousy; the writing the beloved's name everywhere, etc. These alliances are sometimes sexual, but oftener not so—though full of "psychic erethism."

———

In the same Appendix he quotes a woman of thirty-three, who writes, "At fourteen I had my first case of love, but it was with a girl. It was insane, intense love, but had the same quality and sensations as my first love with a man at eighteen. In neither case was the object idealized: I was perfectly aware of their faults; nevertheless, my whole being was lost, immersed, in their existence. The first lasted two years, the second seven years. No love has since been so intense, but now these two persons, though living, are no more to me than the veriest stranger."

———

Another woman of thirty-five writes, "Girls between the ages of fourteen and eighteen at college or girls' schools often fall in love with the same sex. This is not friendship. The loved one is older, more advanced, more charming or beautiful. When I was a freshman in college I knew at least thirty girls who were in love with a senior. Some sought her because it was the fashion, but I knew that my own homage and that of many others was sincere and passionate. I loved her because she was brilliant and utterly indifferent to the love shown her. She was not pretty, though at the time we thought her beautiful. One of her adorers, on being slighted, was ill for two weeks. On her return she was speaking to me when the object of our admiration came into the room. The shock was too great, and she fainted. When I reached the senior year I was the recipient of languishing glances, original verses, roses, and passionate letters written at midnight and three in the morning."

———

"Passionate friendships among girls, from the most innocent to the most elaborate excursions in the direction of Lesbos, are extremely common in theatres, both among actresses, and even more among chorus and ballet-girls."— HAVELOCK ELLIS, "Sexual Inversion," p. 130.

———

"The love of homosexual women is often very passionate, as is that of Urnings. Just like these, the former often feel themselves blessed when they love happily. Nevertheless, to many of them, as to the Urning, is the circumstance very painful that in consequence of their antipathy to the touch of the male they are not in the position to found a family. Sometimes, when the love of a homosexual woman is not responded to, serious disturbances of the nerve-system may ensue, leading even to paroxysms of fury."— A. MOLL, op. cit., p. 338.

———

"It is noteworthy how many inverted women have, with more or less fraud, been married to the woman of their choice, the couple living happily together for long periods. I know of one case, probably unique, in which the ceremony was gone through without any deception on any side; a congenitally inverted English woman of distinguished intellectual ability, now dead, was attached to the wife of a clergyman, who, in full cognisance of all the facts of the case, privately married the two ladies in his own church."—HAVELOCK ELLIS, op. cit., p. 146, footnote.

———

"Seven or eight girls, we are told (in Montaigne's 'Journal du Voyage en Italie,' 1350), belonging to Chaumont, resolved to dress and to work as men; one of these came to Vitry to work as a weaver, and was looked upon as a well-conditioned young man, and liked by everyone. At Vitry she became betrothed to a woman, but, a quarrel arising, no marriage took place. Afterwards, 'she fell in love with a woman whom she married, and with whom she lived for four or five months, to the wife's great contentment, it is said; but having been recognised by some one from Chaumont, and brought to justice, she was condemned to be hanged. She said she would even prefer this to living again as a girl, and was hanged for using illicit inventions to supply the defects of her sex'."—Ibid, p. 119.

———

"It is evident that there must be some radical causes for the frequency of homosexuality among prostitutes. One such cause doubtless lies in the character of the prostitute's relations with men; these relations are of a professional character, and, as the business element becomes emphasized, the possibility of sexual satisfaction diminishes; at the best also there lacks the sense of social equality, the feeling of possession, and scope for the exercise of feminine affection and devotion."—Ibid, p. 149.

———

"Among the inscribed prostitutes of Berlin there are without doubt a great number who honour the love of women. I am told from well- informed sources, that about twenty-five per cent. of the prostitutes of Berlin have relations with other women."—A. MOLL, op. cit., p. 331.

———

"Karl Heinrich Ulrichs (born in 1825 near Aurich), who for many years expounded and defended homosexual love, and whose views are said to have had some influence in drawing Westphal's attention to the matter, was a Hanoverian legal official (Amtsassessor), himself sexually inverted. From 1864 onward, at first under the name of 'Numa Numantius,' and subsequently under his own name, Ulrichs published in various parts of Germany a long series of works dealing with this question, and made various attempts to obtain a revision of the legal position of the sexual invert in Germany.

"Although not a writer whose psychological views can carry much scientific weight, Ulrichs appears to have been a man of most brilliant ability, and his knowledge is said to have been of almost universal extent; he was not only well-versed in his own special subjects of jurisprudence and theology, but in many branches of natural science, as well as in archæology; he was also regarded by many as the best Latinist of his time. In 1880 he left Germany and settled in Naples, and afterwards at Aquila in the Abruzzi, whence he issued a Latin periodical. He died in 1895."—HAVELOCK ELLIS, op. cit., p. 33.

———

Ulrichs enters into an elaborate classification of human types, with a corresponding nomenclature, which, though somewhat ponderous, has been of use. Among males, for instance, he distinguishes the quite normal man, whom he calls "Dioning," from the invert, whom he calls "Urning." Among Urnings, again, he distinguishes (1) those who are thoroughly manly in appearance and in mental habit and character ("Mannlings"), and who tend to love softer and younger specimens of their own sex; (2) those who are effeminate in appearance and cast of mind ("Weiblings"), and who love rougher and older men; and (3) those who are of a medium type ("Zwischen-Urnings") and love young men. Then again there is the "Urano-Dioning," who is born with a capacity of love in both directions, i.e., for women and for men. He is generally of the manly type. And besides these, some sub-species, like the "Uraniaster," who is a normal man who has contracted the Urning habit, and the "Virilised Urning," who is an Urning who has contracted the normal habit, though this is not really natural to him! The whole may be set out in a table as follows:—

The Human Male:
  (a) Normal Man or Dioning—called Uraniaster when he acquires
      Urning tendencies.
  (b) Urning:
    1. Mannling.
    2. Zwischen-Urning.
    3. Weibling.
    4. Also called Virilised Urning when he acquires the normal habit.
  (c) Urano-Dioning.

If we add to this a corresponding table for the female we shall have an idea of the complication of Ulrichs' system! Yet, complex as it is, and whatever criticisms we may make upon it, we must allow that it does not exceed the complexity of the real facts of Nature. (See K. H. ULRICHS' "Memnon," ch. ii.-v.)

———

Krafft-Ebing's analysis of the subject is fully as elaborate as that of Ulrichs. It is given by J. A. SYMONDS in the form of a table, as follows:—

Sexual Inversion
  1. Acquired:
    a) Persistent.
    b) Episodical.
  2. Congenital:
    a) Psychic Hermaphrodites.
    b) Urnings
     i) Male Habitus (Mannlings).
     ii) Female Habitus (Weiblings).
    c) Androgyni.

And Symonds continues:—"What is the rational explanation of the facts presented to us by the analysis which I have formulated in this table, cannot as yet be thoroughly determined. We do not know enough about the law of sex in human beings to advance a theory. Krafft-Ebing and writers of his school are at present inclined to refer them all to diseases of the nervous centres, inherited, congenital, excited by early habits of self-abuse. The inadequacy of this method I have already attempted to set forth; and I have also called attention to the fact that it does not sufficiently account for the phenomena known to us through history and through everyday experience." [It should be noted that in later editions of his book Krafft-Ebing considerably modifies the view that these sex-variations all indicate disease.]—"A Problem in Modern Ethics," p. 46.

———

Moll, speaking of the act so commonly credited to Urnings (sodomy), says:—"The common assumption is that the intercourse of Urnings consists in this. But it is a great error to suppose that this act is so frequent among them."—A. MOLL, op. cit., p. 139.

———

And Krafft-Ebing also speaks of it as rare among true Urnings, though not uncommon among old roués and debauchees of more normal temperament.—"Psychopathia Sexualis," 7th edition, p. 258.

———

"The Urning denies not only the 'unnaturalness' of his leanings, but also their pathological character; he protests against comparison with the lame and the deaf. The occasional coincidence of sexual inversion with other really morbid conditions settles nothing, nor is the reminder that it is antagonistic to the purpose of race-propagation a proof; for who can assure us that Nature has intended all people for race-propagation? Even to the worker-bee Nature has not granted this function, although in her stunted female sex-organs there exists an undeniable indication or suggestion of sex-feeling."— A. MOLL, op. cit., p. 271. (From a letter by a sixty year old Urning.)

———

"Homosexuality, therefore, might be described as an abnormal variety of the sex-impulse, but hardly as a morbid variety. If you like, it might be termed an arrest of development or a kind of reversion. And this is quite in accord with the fact that the best experts in the subject have so far not discovered more psychic abnormalities among homosexuals than among heterosexuals— nor more degeneracy or signs of degeneracy."—Consulting-Physician Dr. PAUL NAECKE, in Der Tag, 26th Oct., 1907.

———

"As a result of these considerations Ulrichs concludes that there is no real ground for the persecution of Urnings except such as may be found in the repugnance felt by the vast numerical majority for an insignificant minority. The majority encourages matrimony, condones seduction, sanctions prostitution, legalises divorce, in the interest of its own sexual proclivities. It makes temporary or permanent unions illegal for the minority whose inversion of instinct it abhors. And this persecution, in the popular mind at any rate, is justified, like many other inequitable acts of prejudice or ignorance, by theological assumptions and the so- called mandates of revelation."—"A Problem in Modern Ethics," p. 83.

———

"We understand by 'homosexual' a person who feels himself drawn to individuals of the same sex by feelings of real love. Whether or not he acts in accordance with this homosexual feeling is, from the scientific standpoint, beside the question. Just as there are normal folk who live chastely, so there are homosexual persons whose love bears a distinctly psychic, ideal and 'platonic' character. . . .

"The feminine impress, in the case of homosexual men, is in general best indicated by the presence of greater sensitiveness and receptivity, also by the dominance of the emotional life, by a strong artistic sense, especially in the direction of music, often too by a tendency to mysticism, and by various inclinations and habits feminine in the good or less good sense of the word. This blending of temperament, however, does not make the homosexual as such a less worthy person. He is indeed not of the same nature as the heterosexual, but he is of equal worth."—Dr. M.

HIRSCHFELD'S evidence as medical specialist in the Moltké-Harden trial.

———

"One serious objection to recognising and tolerating sexual inversion has always been that it tends to check the population. This was a sound political and social argument in the time of Moses, when a small militant tribe needed to multiply to the full extent of its procreative capacity. It is by no means so valid in our age, when the habitable portions of the globe are rapidly becoming overcrowded. Moreover, we must bear in mind that society under the existing order sanctions female prostitution, whereby men and women, though normally procreative, are sterilized to an indefinite extent."—J. A. SYMONDS, "A Problem in Modern Ethics," p. 82.

———

"Before Justinian, both Constantine and Theodosius passed laws against sexual inversion, committing the offenders to 'avenging flames.' But these statutes were not rigidly enforced, and modern opinion on the subject may be said to flow from Justinian's legislation. Opinion, in matters of custom and manners, always follows law. Though Imperial edicts could not eradicate a passion which is inherent in human nature, they had the effect of stereotyping extreme punishments in all the codes of Christian nations, and of creating a permanent social antipathy."— Ibid, p. 13.

———

"Our modern attitude is sometimes traced back to the Jewish Law and its survival in St. Paul's opinion on this matter. But the Jewish Law itself had a foundation. Wherever the enlargement of the population becomes a strongly-felt social need—as it was among the Jews in their exaltation of family life, and as it was when the European populations were constituted—there homosexuality has been regarded as a crime, even punishable with death. . . . It was in the fourth century at Rome that the strong modern opposition to it was formulated in law. The Roman race had long been decaying; sexual perversions of all kinds flourished; the population was dwindling. At the same time Christianity with its Judaic-Pauline antagonism to homosexuality was rapidly spreading. The statesmen of the day, anxious to quicken the failing pulses of national life, utilised this powerful Christian feeling. Constantine, Theodosius, Valentinian, all passed laws against homosexuality—the last, at all events, ordaining as a penalty the vindices flammæ."—HAVELOCK ELLIS, op. cit., p. 206.

———

"At the present time, shoemakers, who make shoes to measure, deal more rationally with individuals than our teachers and schoolmasters do, in their application to moral principles. The sexually intermediate forms of individuals are treated exactly as if they were good examples of the ideal male or female types. There is wanted an 'orthopædic' treatment of the soul, instead of the torture caused by the application of ready-made conventional shapes. The present system stamps out much that is original, uproots much that is truly natural, and distorts much into artificial and unnatural forms."—O. WEININGER, "Sex and Character," ch. v.

———

"What is new in my view is that according to it homosexuality cannot be regarded as an atavism or as due to arrested embryonic development, or to incomplete differentiation of sex; it cannot be regarded as an anomaly of rare occurrence interpolating itself in customary complete separation of the sexes. Homosexuality is merely the sexual condition of those intermediate sexual forms that stretch from one ideal sexual condition to the other ideal sexual condition. In my view, all actual organisms have both homosexuality and heterosexuality."—O. WEININGER, "Sex and Character," ch. iv.

———

"How is it then that in our age reputed so philanthropic, whole classes of men, on account of inborn mental abnormalities, are marked down and banned, frantically persecuted, publicly branded, and threatened with the severest legal penalties? Any one would hardly believe what gross cases of justiciary murder, morally speaking, still take place in this matter even at the end of the nineteenth century. To the pitiful ignorance of the judges, to the thousand inherited prejudices of public opinion, as well as to the mental slavery of legislative bodies, must it be ascribed that the penal code of most civilised states is still in great measure formulated in the gloomy spirit of the Middle Ages."— O. de Joux, "Die Enterbten des Liebesglückes," p. 16.

———

"Up till now homosexual humanity has found itself in a peculiar position. Its mouth was closed, it could not speak. It was bound hand and foot and could not move. But now there has come an important change. Science has taken the part of these folk and defended their honour . . . I protest therefore earnestly that these men, whether by means of the Law or any other means, should no longer be branded in the name of Christianity."—From a letter written by a Catholic priest in reply to a circular sent by the Humane-Science Committee of Berlin. (See "Jahrbuch der Sexuellen Zwischenstufen," vol. ii., p. 177.)

———

"Thus the very basest of all trades, that of chantage [blackmailing] is encouraged by the law. . . . The miserable persecuted wretch, placed between the alternative of paying money down or of becoming socially impossible, losing a valued position, and seeing dishonour burst upon himself and family, pays; and still the more he pays the greedier becomes the vampire who sucks his life-blood, until at last there lies nothing else before him except total financial ruin or disgrace. Who will be astonished if the nerves of an individual in this position are not equal to the horrid strain? In some cases the nerves give way altogether. . . . Alter the law and instead of increasing vice you will diminish it. The temptation to ply a disgraceful profession with the object of extorting money would be removed."—"A Problem in Modern Ethics," pp. 56 and 86.

———

"You will rightly infer that it is difficult for me to say exactly how I regard (morally) the homosexual tendency. Of this much, however, I am certain: that even if it were possible I would not exchange my inverted nature for a normal one. I suspect that the sexual emotions and even inverted ones have a more subtle significance than is generally attributed to them;

but modern moralists either fight shy of transcendental interpretations or see none, and I am ignorant and unable to solve the mystery these feelings seem to imply."— HAVELOCK ELLIS, op. cit., p. 65, "case" ix.

———

"I cannot regard my sexual feelings as unnatural or abnormal, since they have disclosed themselves so perfectly naturally and spontaneously within me. All that I have read in books or heard spoken about the ordinary sexual love, its intensity and passion, life-long devotion, love at first sight, etc., seems to me to be easily matched by my own experiences in homosexual form; and with regard to the morality of this complex subject, my feeling is that it is the same as should prevail in love between man and woman, namely: that no bodily satisfaction should be sought at the cost of another person's distress or degradation. I am sure that this kind of love is, notwithstanding the physical difficulties that attend it, as deeply stirring and ennobling as the other kind, if not more so; and I think that for a perfect relationship the actual sex-gratifications (whatever they may be) probably hold a less important place in this love than in the other."—Ibid, "case" vii., p. 58.

———

"I grew older, I entered my professional studies, and I was very diligent with them. I lived in a great capital, I moved much in general society. I had a large and lively group of friends. But always, over and over, I realised that, in the kernel, at the very root and fibre of myself, there was the throb and glow, the ebb and the surge, the seeking as in a vain dream to realise again that passion of friendship which could so far transcend the cold modern idea of the tie; the Over-Friendship, the Love-Friendship of Hellas, which meant that between man and man could exist—the sexual-psychic love. That was still possible! I knew that now. I had read it in the verses or the prose of the Greek or Latin or Oriental authors who have written out every shade of its beauty or unloveliness, its worth or debasement— from Theokritos to Martial, or Abu-Nuwas, to Platen, Michel Angelo, Shakespeare. I had learned it from the statues of sculptors—in those lines so often vivid with a merely physical male beauty—works which beget, which sprang from, the sense of it in a race. I had half-divined it in the music of a Beethoven and a Tschaikowsky before knowing facts in the life-stories of either of them—or of an hundred other tone- autobiographists. And I had recognised what it all meant to most people to-day—from the disgust, scorn, and laughter of my fellow- men when such an emotion was hinted at."—Imre: a memorandum, by XAVIER MAYNE, p. 110. Naples, R. Rispoli, 1906.

"Presently, during that same winter, accident opened my eyes wider to myself. Since then, I have needed no further knowledge from the Tree of my Good and Evil. I met with a mass of serious studies, German, Italian, French, English, from the chief European specialists and theorists on the similisexual topic; many of them with quite other views than those of my well-meaning but far too conclusive Yankee doctor (who had recommended marriage as a cure). I learned of the much-discussed theories of 'secondary sexes' and 'intersexes.' I learned of the theories and facts of homosexualism, of the Uranian Love, of the Uranian race, of the 'Sex within a Sex.' . . . I came to know their enormous distribution all over the world to-day; and of the grave attention that European scientists and jurists have been devoting to problems concerned with homosexualism. I could pursue intelligently the growing efforts to set right the public mind as to so ineradicable and misunderstood a phase of humanity. I realised that I had always been a member of that hidden brotherhood and Sub-Sex, or Super-Sex. In wonder too I informed myself of its deep instinctive freemasonries—even to organised ones—in every social class, every land, and every civilisation."—Ibid, pp. 134, 135.

"Thus in sexual inversion we have what may be fairly called a 'sport' or variation, one of those organic aberrations which we see throughout living nature, in plants and in animals." . . . "All these organic variations which I have here mentioned to illustrate sexual inversion, are abnormalities. It is important that we should have a clear idea as to what abnormality is. Many people imagine that what is abnormal is necessarily diseased.

That is not the case, unless we give the word disease an inconveniently and illegitimately wide extension. It is both inconvenient and inexact to speak of colour-blindness, criminality and genius as diseases in the same sense as we speak of scarlet fever, tuberculosis, or general paralysis as diseases."—HAVELOCK ELLIS, op. cit., p. 186.

———

"I have had for some time past a theory about this 'Homogenic' business—I do not suppose it is new—but it is that when man reaches a certain stage of development and approaches the totality of Human Nature, there gets to exist in him, though subordinately at first, a female element as well as a male. That is to say that as he passes the various barriers, he passes the barrier of sex too, on his way to become the complete Human—the Universal."—From a private letter.

———

"Great geniuses, men like Goethe, Shakespeare, Shelley, Byron, Darwin, all had the feminine soul very strongly developed in them. . . . As we are continually meeting in cities women who are one-quarter, or one-eighth, or so on, MALE . . . so there are in the Inner Self similar half-breeds, all adapting themselves to circumstances with perfect ease. The Greeks recognised that such a being could exist even in harmony with Nature, and so beautified and idealised it as Sappho."—CHARLES G. LELAND, "The Alternate Sex," pp. 41 and 57. London, 1904.

———

"I have considered and inquired into this question for many years; and it has long been my settled conviction that no breach of morality is involved in homosexual love; that, like every other passion, it tends, when duly understood and controlled by spiritual feeling, to the physical and moral health of the individual and the race, and that it is only its brutal perversions which are immoral. I have known many persons more or less the subjects of this passion, and I have found them a particularly high-minded, upright, refined, and (I must add) pure-minded class of men."—Communicated by Professor —— in Appendix to HAVELOCK ELLIS'S "Sexual Inversion," p. 240.

―――

"What from the beginning struck me most, but now appears perfectly clear and indeed necessary is that among the homosexuals there is found the MOST remarkable class of men, namely, those whom I call SUPERVIRILE. These men stand by virtue of the special variation of their soul-material, just as much above Man, as the normal sex man does above Woman. Such an individual is able to bewitch men by his soul-aroma, as they—though passively—bewitch him. But as he always lives in men's society, and men, so to speak, sit at his feet, it comes about that such a supervirile often climbs the very highest steps of spiritual evolution, of social position, and of manly capacity. Hence it arises that the most famous names of the world and the history of culture stand rightly or wrongly on the list of homosexuals. Names like Alexander the Great, Socrates, Plato, Julius Cæsar, Michel-Angelo, Charles XII. of Sweden, William of Orange, and so forth. Not only is this so, but it must be so. As certainly as a woman's hero remains a spiritually inferior man, must a man's hero—well BE a man's hero, if in any way he has the stuff for it.

"Consequently the German penal code, in stamping homosexuality as a crime, puts the highest blossoms of humanity on the proscription list."— Professor Dr. JAEGER, "Die Entdeckung der Seele," pp. 268, 269.

―――

"The licentious or garrulous or morbid types of inverts have been so honoured with publicity that the other types are even yet little known. The latter, in the maturity of their intellectual and moral nature, cease to look upon sex as the pivot of the universe. They cease to repine about their lot. They have their mission to fulfil here below, and they try to fulfil it as best they can. In the same way we find there are heterosexual (or normal) folk who at a certain stage of their growth free themselves from the sexual life."—M. A. RAFFALOVICH, "Uranisme et Unisexualité," p. 74.

―――

"The well-bred, highly-cultured Urning is a complete Idealist; matter is for him only a symbol of thought, and the actual only the living expression of the Invisible."—DE JOUX, "Die Enterbten des Liebesglückes," p. 46.

———

"As nature and social law are so cruel as to impose a severe celibacy on him his whole being is consequently of astonishing freshness and superb purity, and his manners of life modest as those of a saint—a thing which, in the case of a man in blooming health and moving about in the world, is certainly very unusual."— Ibid, p. 41.

———

"If the soul of woman in its usual form represents a secret closed with seven seals, it is—when prisoned in the sturdy body of a man and fused with some of the motives of manhood, a far more enigmatic scripture of whose sibylline meaning one can never be really sure. Only the Urning can understand the Urning."—Ibid, p. 63.

———

"Because they (Urnings) themselves are of a very complex nature and put together of opposing elements, they seek out and love the simple, plain, and straightforward natures. Because they continually suffer from the rebellion of their desires against good taste and morals, they often long for a barbaric freedom. And because their every emotion is cut short, distracted, and worn out by the thousand doubts and suspicions of their Urning-minds, they gather to themselves men who are wont to live straight from feeling to action, and who work from untamed masterly instincts, as sure as the animals."—Ibid, p. 97.

———

"It is true that we are often inferior to normal men in force of will, worldly wisdom, and sense of duty; but on the other hand, in depth and delicacy of feeling and every virtue of the heart, we are far superior. We cannot LOVE women, but we lament with them, and help them on the hearth and by the cradle, in need and loneliness, as their most unselfish friends . . . We do not despise women because they are weak, for we are much clearer-sighted, much less prejudiced than the so-called lords of creation, much nobler, more helpful, and just-minded than they. . . . Anyhow, if either of the sexes has cause to withhold its respect in any degree from the other—which has the most cause? Say what you will of them, the second and third sexes—women and Urnings—are ever so much better than the brutal egotistical Men, who to-day are plunged in grossest materialism; for, with whatever corruption, both the former are still of purer heart, easier kindled towards whatever is good, and more capable of genuine enthusiasm and love of their fellows, than the latter."—Ibid, p. 204.

———

"Embodying as he does Love, Patience, Renunciation, Humility and Mildness, the Urning should seek to soothe with his gentle hand all hurts, and to heal all wounds, which are the results of weak Man's original sinfulness. The tender emotions in his breast, his all too soft and easily troubled heart, his delicate sensitiveness and receptiveness of all that is lofty and pure, his mildness, goodness and inexhaustible patience—all these divine gifts of his soul point clearly to the conclusion that the great framer of the world meant to create in Urnings a noble priesthood, a race of Samaritans, a severely pure order of men, in order to offer a strong counterpoise to the immoral tendencies of the human race, which increase with its increasing culture."—Ibid, p. 253.

———

"When I review the cases I have brought forward and the mental history of the inverted I have known, I am inclined to say that if we can enable an invert to be healthy, self-restrained and self- respecting, we have often done better than to convert him to the mere feeble simulacrum of a normal man. An appeal to the paiderastia of the best Greek days, and the dignity, temperance, even chastity, which it involved, will sometimes find a ready response in the emotional enthusiastic nature of the congenital invert. The 'manly' love celebrated by Walt Whitman in 'Leaves of Grass,' although it may be of more doubtful value for general use, furnishes a wholesome and robust ideal to the invert who is insensitive to normal ideals. It is by some such method of self-treatment as this that most of the more highly intelligent men and women whose histories I have already briefly recorded have at last slowly and instinctively reached a condition of relative health and peace, physical and moral."—HAVELOCK ELLIS, "Sexual Inversion," p. 202.

———

"From America a lady writes:—'Inverts should have the courage and independence to be themselves, and to demand an investigation. If one strives to live honourably, and considers the greatest good to the greatest number, it is not a crime nor a disgrace to be an invert. I do not need the law to defend me, neither do I desire to have any concessions made for me, nor do I ask my friends to sacrifice their ideals for me. I too have ideals which I shall always hold. All that I desire—and I claim it as my right—is the freedom to exercise this divine gift of loving, which is not a menace to society nor a disgrace to me. Let it once be understood that the average invert is not a moral degenerate nor a mental degenerate, but simply a man or a woman who is less highly specialised, less completely differentiated, than other men and women, and I believe the prejudice against them will disappear, and if they live uprightly they will surely win the esteem and consideration of all thoughtful people. I know what it is to be an invert—who feels himself set apart from the rest of mankind—to find one human heart who trusts him and understands him, and I know how almost impossible this is, and will be, until the world is made aware of these facts.'"—Ibid, p. 213.

CPSIA information can be obtained at www.ICGtesting.com

235174LV00001B/5/A

9 781406 823813